Taste
of 1001 nights

Mahshid Babzartabi

First published by Busybird Publishing 2022

Copyright © 2022 Mahshid Babzartabi

ISBN:
Hardcover Print: 978-1-922691-71-2
Ebook: 978-1-922691-72-9

This work is copyright. Apart from any use permitted under the *Copyright Act 1968*, no part of this publication may be reproduced, stored in a retrieval system or transmitted in any form or by any means, electronic, mechanical, photocopying, recording or otherwise, without the prior written permission of Mahshid Babzartabi.

The information in this book is based on the author's experiences and opinions. The author and publisher disclaim responsibility for any adverse consequences, which may result from use of the information contained herein. Permission to use any external content has been sought by the author. Any breaches will be rectified in further editions of the book.

Cover design: Busybird Publishing

Layout and typesetting: Busybird Publishing

Photography: Mahshid Babzartabi, Gigi Jafari, Raheleh Rezaei, Faeezeh Rafati, Mamma Shookoh catering, Shahnaz Daghagheleh, Neda Bazyariyan, Azadeh Arzhangi

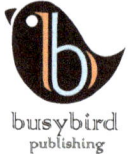

Busybird Publishing
2/118 Para Road
Montmorency, Victoria
Australia 3094
www.busybird.com.au

This book speaks of home, speaks of love and is presented to the love of my life, my beloved late son Masoud.

For all those dishes that I cooked from the bottom of my heart, every single time I wished you were there and could taste it.

All these years, I just imagined, you're at school and I'm cooking for you, like the old days.

When you're back home from school, mommy made your favourite dish and it's ready on the table. Till then.

Contents

Introduction	1

Teahouse food — 7

Persian tomato omelette	11
Eshkeneh	15
Adasi	19
Abgosht	23
Gaghour Baghour, or Hasrat O Al Molok	27

Street food — 31

Sosis Bandari	35
Samosa	39
Falafel	45
Kabab Loghmeh	49
Laboo (hot beetroots in syrup)	53
Baghali (hot broad beans)	57
Yeralma Yumurta (boiled potato and egg)	61

Local food — 65

Ash-e Doogh (thin yogurt soup)	67
Zeytoon parvardeh (processed olive from North of Iran)	71
Mirza Ghasemi (smoked eggplant with garlic and egg)	77
Akbar Joheh (Akbar chicken)	81
Kofteh tabrizi (juicy meatballs with herbs and lentil)	85
Ghalyeh Mahi (fried fish stew in tamarind sauce)	91
Gheymeh Nesar (or jewelled rice)	95
Tas Kabab	101

Food for special religious or national occasions — 105

Halva	107
Ash-E-Shoo-Le- Ghalam Kar	111
Ash-e-Ash-E-Reshteh (Persian noodle soup)	119
Shoo Le Zard (saffron rice pudding)	127
Adas polo (green lentils and rice with minced meat and raisins)	131
Sabzi Polo Mahi (cooked rice with herbs and fried fish)	135
Saffron drink with basil seed and rose water	143

Food kids love — 147

Istanbuli polo	149
Loobiya Polo	151
Kotlet (Persian patties)	155

Food with medical benefits — 159

Kachi	161
Chickpea soup	165
Harireh badam (silky almond meal)	169

Food for weddings and formal ceremonies — 171

Zereshk Polo Morgh (chicken barberry and saffron rice	175
Baghali Polo (lamb shank with rice and broad beans and dill)	179
Gheymeh & Ghoormeh	185
Ghoormeh Sabzi (a classic traditional lamb and herb stew)	191
Tah-Dig and Tah-Chin	197
Fesenjoon	203
Tah-Chin	209

Thank you — 216

Introduction

According to a legendary tale, Iran, also called Persia, used to be called the land of 1001 nights. In this epic story, there was a beautiful, defiant girl called Shahrzad, whose father was one of the king's ministers.

Looking for revenge on his late wife, who had betrayed him, the king married a virgin girl every night, and the day after his marriage, ordered his executioner to behead his one-night bride.

It was the minister's mission to find virgin girls for the king, but no one wanted to be a queen for only one night, only to be executed the day after.

While everyone was ruled to obey the king, no one in court could find a solution for these unlucky marriages until Shahrzad told her father that she had the solution for this problem, and asked to be allowed to marry the king. But the minister adored his daughter, and couldn't let the king kill her.

Shahrzad kept insisting until she convinced her father she would be safe at the end. She assured her father she could do something that would stop the king revenging and taking his anger out on virgin girls.

Not a very pleasant story, but that's how Iran ended up being called the land of 1001 nights, so listen to the rest of the story to find out why.

On the first night of her marriage, Shahrzad started telling a story for the king. She was a great storyteller and the king was so eager to hear the story but it was too long to be finished in one night. So she said to the king, 'It's too late and we're both too tired. Let me leave the rest of the story to tomorrow night.'

Every night before Shahrzad finished a story, she started another story, the rest of which needed to be left for the night after.

It took 1001 nights for Shahrzad to run out of stories to tell the king.

On the night when the last story was told, the king asked interestedly, eagerly for another story, but Shahrzad said she didn't know any other story. Her stories were finished and it was time for the king to order her execution.

But the king had become used to Shahrzad's stories and her pleasant presence every night. He didn't want to lose her and 1001 nights was enough time for him to fall in love with her.

Since there was no addictive media back then, such stories were not only interesting but would give other nations a hint of what was happening on other sides of the world. This is the reason Iran used to be called the land of 1001 nights.

A lot of people are also confused about whether they should call the country Iran or Persia and the reason is that before Arabs invaded Iran, it used to be called Persia. When Arabs invaded and forced the country to change its Zartostian religion to Islam, they gave this country the new name of Iran.

I have faced many people who don't know much about my homeland and they are always confused between these two names, but both are pointing to the same land.

Iran, or Persia, or the land of 1001 nights, is a country in southwest Asia: a mountainous, arid, and ethnically diverse country. A country with rich history, famous for its hospitality, fascinating carpets, luxurious caviar, and the best saffron in the world. A country known for lots of reasons, yet not known for the best reason of all, which is Iranian cuisines.

Since all the world's attention has been driven to Iran's political situations, the world doesn't know enough about Persian food. With so much negative propaganda in the media, people only hear the unattractive side of the Iranian story, and its attractions are hidden from view.

It seems the world hasn't spent enough time to discover the best of Iran, including its fascinatingly delicious cuisines.

With a lot of similarity to cuisines across Asia and the Middle East, Iranian food has its own signature taste and stories.

Introduction

Although still considered to be Asian food, Persian food is free from hot and spicy tastes. With the right balance and successful marriage among its ingredients, it is food that gives comfort.

You can feel the right limitation in its spices but the taste of used spices in food are enough to give you a flavour you're looking for in a plate.

Taking advantage of a rich and illustrious history that spans thousands of years, and being in the heart of the well-known Silk Road, brings a huge variety of influences and backstories to Iranian cuisine.

As travellers and merchants started passing by the silky way, they also brought a lot of new tastes and ingredients, such as noodles from China and rice from India, to traditional Persian food. Noodles were not as popular as rice and their special taste meant they were only chosen for some special kinds of soups.

But for rice, the story was different.

The Northern territory of Iran had a wet, humid climate, with lots of rain, which was very good weather to cultivate rice. Gradually, rice became the dominant, preferred dish on Iranian tables.

It's called Berenj (be = with and renj or ranj = suffer) since the process to cultivate and harvest rice was very time consuming, needing strong levels of effort and it was only with lots of hardship and suffering that farmers could get their hands on the final product of white rice (brown rice was never popular on Iranian tables, until recently when people started being more aware about health issues).

This long and hard process made rice even more expensive than anyone could afford to have it as a daily food. So almost 100 years ago, when agriculture was not still mechanised, it was not common to have rice as much as we have it these days. I heard from my grandmother that they would only have rice once a year, on New Year's night.

Going back further to the Safavi dynasty, nearly 500 years ago, a lot of changes happened in all aspects of Persian life, including in people's eating habits.

It was then that there was a huge rise in the popularity of rice across Iran, but still only the rich could afford to have it every day.

Nowadays, people in Iran eat rice at least once a day, mostly for lunch.

The variety of rice dishes is so big that there are enough options for every taste. Most of these varieties come to the table with a huge range of different, usually meat, stews called khoresht, eaten as the main dish.

Khoresht, coming from the word khordan (meaning to eat), and the meaning of something you eat with rice, is always served with saffron rice.

Food has an important role in Iranian culture and social communications.

As older Iranians believe, where you eat is a holy place and where you receive blessings. So, in many states of Iran, food has more meaning than just eating – sometimes it is considered as a holy and religious practice.

That's why there are some special dishes only produced to be used in religious ceremonies. Some of these special dishes carry their culture and traditional stories behind them.

For each region of Iran, anything related to food culture is more definitive than what you simply see in a dish. Food culture is a national heritage that carries a country's traditions; the historical, cultural, and religious signs of a land; along with stories about that dish. Food is a meaningful cultural activity that relays social relationships.

The huge ethnic diversity across a number of regions, along with widespread geography, is a cause for the great variety of cuisine in Iran.

This variety follows each region's climate, culture, traditions, and lifestyle, but while the availability of different foods colours a region's table, dishes are not limited by simplicity most of the time.

You could even say that each state's eating habits are a cultural show to express how advanced that region is compared to others.

In this book you will not only discover recipes for some of the most well-known Persian dishes, we will travel together to the heart of each cuisine's backstory. My main focus will be on very traditional cuisines, their origins, and the stories behind them. If you ask an expert what the most famous Persian foods are, you may not be able to find all of their answers in here, but you will definitely be introduced to some recipes with mesmerising stories behind them. Beyond a collection of recipes, this book is an introduction to the tradition and culture of a nation that hasn't been introduced to and appreciated by the world in the right way. Because that is the magic of food: to bring reconciliation between a country and the rest of the world that is trapped in the negativity of propaganda.

Writing this book is breaking my current limitations. I'm banned from travelling to my home due to the current political situation ruling in my country but by sharing these stories and recipes with you, it's possible again.

Come, travel with me to the land of 1001 nights, where for each night there is a cuisine and a story.

Teahouse food

Like most Asian countries, Iran has teahouses, but the real style of old-fashioned teahouses is not available in most parts of the country anymore. All new styles are renovated, modern teahouses to attract more customers which in reality, are very different from what teahouses used to look like.

The real Iranian style of a teahouse – I mean the old fashioned one – is rare, but you may be able to find them in downtown of cities or in regional and remote villages.

Teahouses began to be popular nearly 500 years ago during the Safavi dynasty, when one of the most advanced court families was ruling in Iran. This family brought a lot of changes to the country, including in people's food habits. This is when modernisation started in the country, as Iran started having more political relationships with European countries, sending ambassadors and opening its borders to travellers.

European travellers who came to Iran during that time have written about places for people to socialise, called teahouses, in their books.

In the beginning, teahouses were only open to people from the highest social class. They served different kinds of drinks made from local herbs and sometimes coffee. Tea was not common then so they used to call these places coffee houses.

In the king's court there were special teahouses only for the king and his guests. Working in the teahouses in the king's court was considered to be one of the highest positions in society.

Gradually, socialising in teahouses found its way outside of court, but teahouses were still only open to people from the higher social classes and positions.

But soon, ordinary people had the chance to have their own teahouses. Still, teahouses were only open to men. On rare occasions these days some of the traditional teahouses in regional and remote villages still do not allow women in, but modern teahouses in cities are now more like restaurants and open to all sorts of customers.

Soon, teahouses were everywhere throughout the country, even in villages.

The teahouse was a place for men to be entertained and rest, regardless of all daily routine jobs and activities.

Teahouses would open very early in the morning after daily prayers, since the majority of people in society were Muslim and would pray before sunrise every day.

Obviously being open early in the morning means serving breakfast to customers too.

Besides a normal, routine breakfast which was always freshly baked bread with cheese, butter, honey, jam and heavy cream, teahouses would serve something special too – something that would belong only to that teahouse, like a signature dish. It was then that teahouses' special menus were invented.

Some dishes of this menu were taken from traditional village or street food and some were just invented by the teahouse owners, like Persian tomato omelette, which is still called teahouse omelette.

Teahouses would have three different menus for breakfast, lunch, and dinner.

Breakfast customers were normally every man in the neighbourhood, especially those who left the house very early and didn't have time for breakfast at home.

Less commonly, teahouses would also serve herbal tea called Gool Gave Zabon (borage tea).

Lunch and dinner customers, however, were usually a bit different – either those who were single with no one to cook for them at home, or those who were very much fans of the teahouse's food.

When women found out that their men were so interested in teahouse food, they started to follow their recipes, since women in earlier generations enjoyed nothing more than pleasing their men.

Nowadays, you can hardly find such traditional teahouses, as they have all been renovated into modern style teahouses, which are far different from the original ones. Although these modern teahouses, with lots of heavy traditional decorations and furniture, are beautiful, they are nothing like how teahouses looked in the beginning. In these new teahouses, which are more like restaurants, the menus are completely different, with big menus full of much heavier foods.

Old teahouses used to have only a few dishes on their menu, and customers didn't expect more.

By dinner time, although teahouses were open until midnight, they didn't have as many customers as the rest of the day. So, to attract more customers in the evening, they entertained their customers with games and special theatre, a show with only two actors called teahouses theatre. The shows were all about reading old historic stories and myths in a poetic way, with a special curtain hanging on the wall, with pictures of each character in the poems being read. One person was responsible for reading the poems, and the other would ask him questions about the characters to make their audience better understand the story. Usually, after the storytelling was finished, the second part of the entertainment, which was games, was started. The games were designed for all sorts of customers to get involved at the same time but they were also limited as there was often not enough space in the teahouse. Later, the games turned into a sort of gambling, and this became another reason for more customers to visit teahouses at night.

Now, let's have a look at some teahouse recipes. Here we are going to have recipes for two breakfasts, one lunch, and two dinners that used to be served in teahouses before they turned to the style we see today.

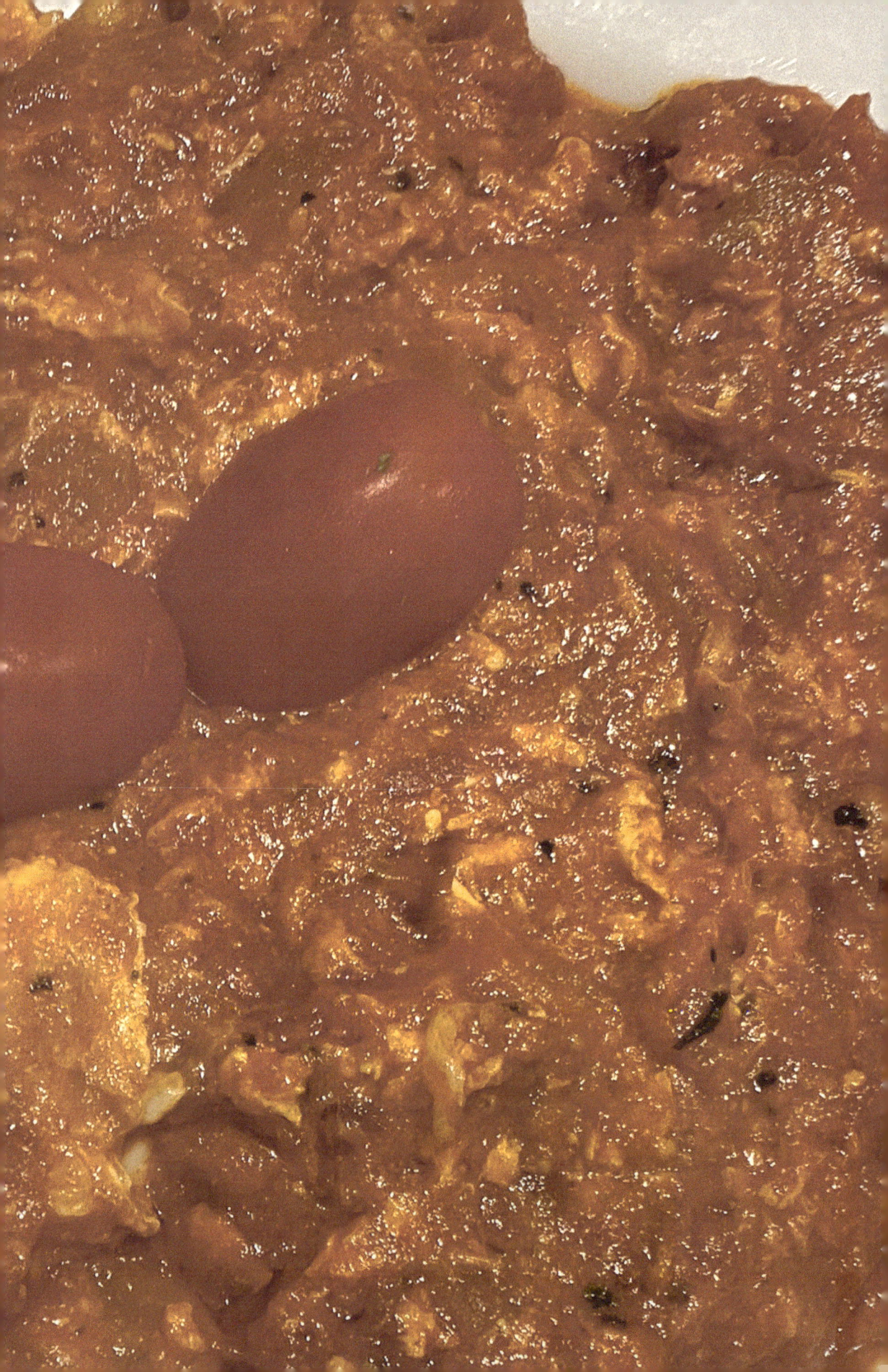

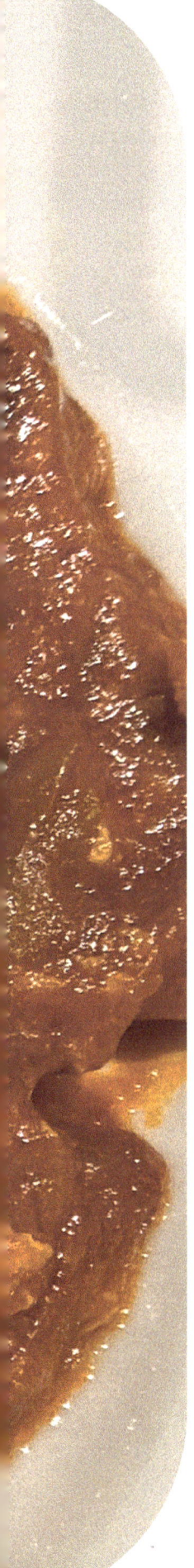

Persian tomato omelette

Probably the most famous Persian teahouse food is teahouse omelette.

When people want give credit to a cook that has prepared Persian tomato omelette at home, they will proudly say, 'Oh it tastes like a teahouse omelette!'

It's also a food for when you don't have enough time, or you're not lucky enough to have a cook next to you, since it's super easy and fast to prepare with simple and limited ingredients: tomato, eggs, butter, salt, pepper, and fried onion.

Some teahouses used to be in remote areas or on out-of-town roads where only passengers would pass by, and while they usually had enough eggs, it was not always easy to get hold of fresh tomatoes, especially in cold seasons. So they started using tomato paste instead of fresh tomatoes and they found out it was even more tasty with tomato paste.

This method and recipe were always in Iranian culture, but the name of omelette was taken from the French omelette, which has its own story. When Napoleon Bonaparte, with his tired and hungry soldiers, was passing by the city of Bessières in southern France, he decided to have a rest. He stopped by an inn and the innkeeper prepared him what is today called an omelette, as it was the fastest and easiest thing he could prepare. Napoleon liked it so much he asked the innkeeper to go to the village and ask everyone to bring him ingredients so he can prepare the whole army the same food.

Since then, people in Bessières cook a giant omelette once a year and feed the whole city with a big ceremony. With the Persian omelette, the story was different – they already had this simple recipe in their menu, but changed the name when they heard Napoleon's omelette story. The Persian recipe is also a bit different from what is called omelette by the rest of the world.

Serves 3

Prep time: 20 minutes

- 1 tbsp butter or vegetable oil
- 1 large onion, finely chopped
- 1 tsp turmeric
- 3 medium tomatoes, washed and diced, or 1 1/2 tbsp tomato paste
- 3 eggs
- salt and black pepper

Method

Fry the onion in the butter in a medium frying pan on a medium heat. As the colour starts to change, add the turmeric and continue to fry for few more minutes.

Add the tomatoes to the fried onion, and continue to cook until almost 80% of the liquid from the tomato is evaporated. If making teahouse omelette, replace the fresh tomato with tomato paste. In this case, you only need to fry the tomato paste for a few seconds before adding the eggs. This stage is very important because, if left too long, the tomato paste will burn and end up giving a dark colour to your omelette.

Break the eggs into the pan and stir for few minutes until the eggs start to thicken.

When the eggs are almost cooked, add salt and pepper to taste.

Serve with Lebanese flatbread, and with sliced fresh onion, if you like.

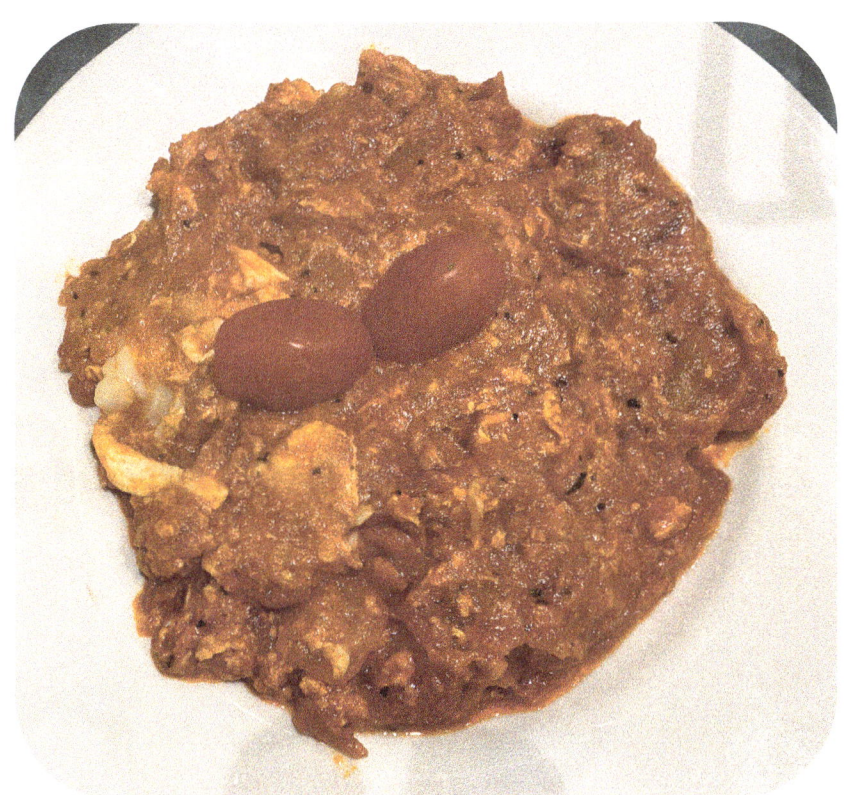

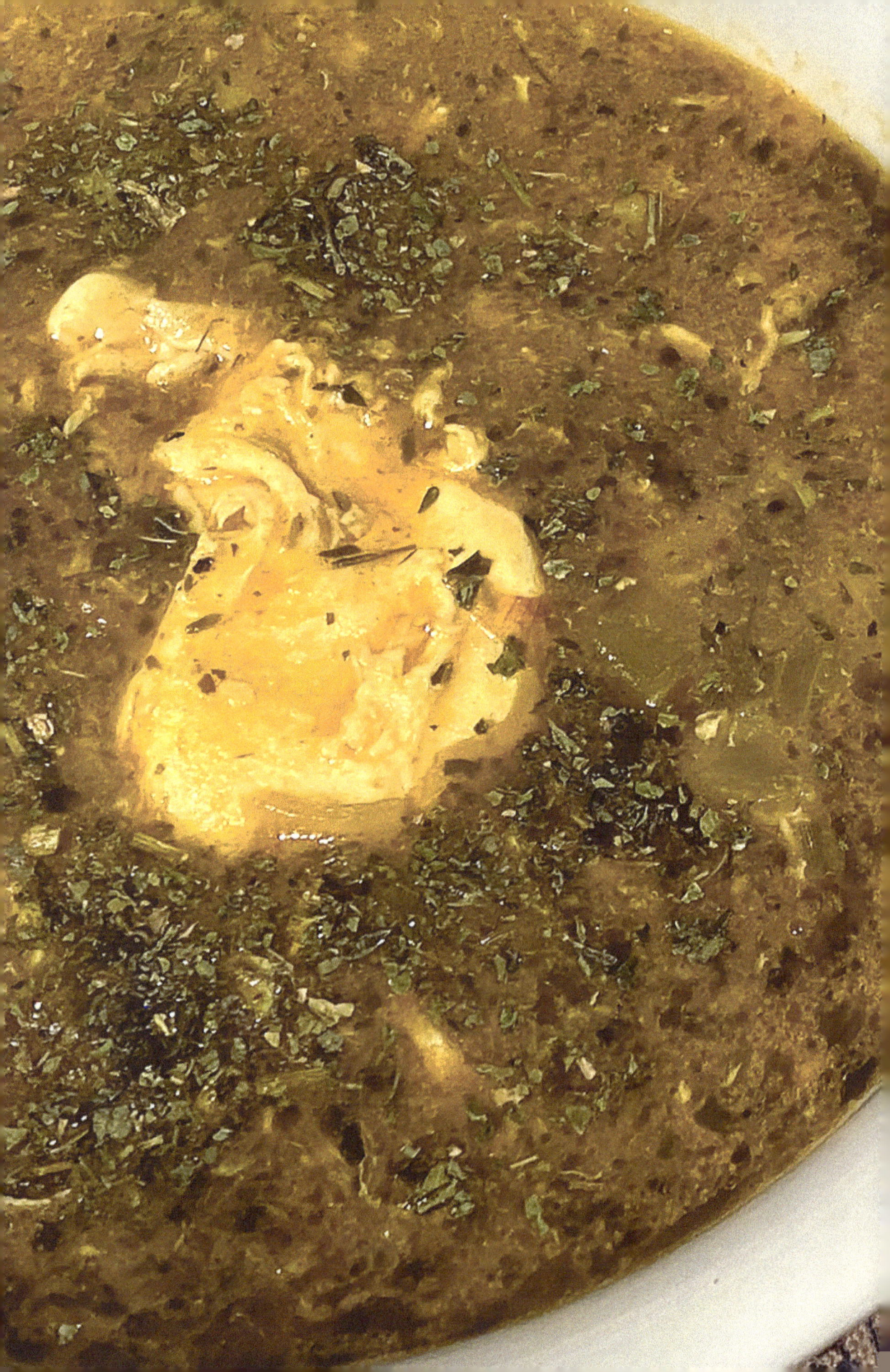

Eshkeneh

Eshkeneh is a quick, nutritious soup originally from the northeast states in Persia. Though it is now known as a teahouse food, it also used to be cooked in villages when both men and women used to work in farms together. By the evening, when they would come back home after a long day, the women of the house, who were responsible for feeding their families, were usually tired with not much time to cook. So Eshkeneh was a great, filling option made from with simple ingredients.

In the old days, when transportation systems were not as advanced as today, people used to cook with whatever they had available. Almost everybody grew their own vegetables in their backyards. Houses used to be big enough that they could keep chooks and in some bigger houses, which looked like farms, people had livestock such as sheep and cows.

Eshkeneh should be eaten with small, broken pieces of bread. These are soaked in the soup when it's served and, once the bread starts to soften, it's topped either with fresh herbs or with broken pieces of onion or pickles in winter. When it was not easy to access fresh herbs, pickle was most of the time considered to be the winter side dish.

Eshkeneh is usually considered a main dish, mostly served in winter, but in teahouses it's usually served as breakfast. Persian people believe having a breakfast like this keeps you energised for the whole day.

Like most other Persian foods, every state has their own recipe for Eshkeneh but some ingredients, such as egg, are found in all versions. The most common and easiest recipe is considered a favourite teahouse food. In some states, Eshkeneh may come with different herbs or extra ingredients.

Serves 2

Prep time: 10 minutes
Cooking time: 30 minutes

- vegetable oil
- 1 large onion, chopped
- 1 tsp turmeric
- salt and black pepper to taste
- 2 tbsp fresh mint, chopped, or 1/2 tbsp dried mint
- 2 tbsp fresh fenugreek, chopped, or 1/2 tbsp dried fenugreek
- 1 tbsp tomato paste
- 2 tbsp pomegranate molasses (optional, to give a sour taste – a common taste in most Persian dishes)
- 2 medium potatoes, diced
- 3 cups water or stock
- 2 eggs
- flatbread, to serve
- spring onion, red radishes, tarragon, and coriander, or fresh onion and pickles to serve

Method

Heat vegetable oil in a medium pan and fry chopped onion until it turns a golden caramelised colour.

When the onion turns golden, add the turmeric, salt, and pepper and stir.

Add the fresh or dried mint and fenugreek and stir.

Add the tomato paste and pomegranate molasses and stir.

Add the diced potato, stir then add the water and bring to the boil. When the water is boiling, cover the pot with a lid and reduce the heat to a simmer for 20 minutes.

Crack the eggs into the pot. Stir the mixture to scramble the eggs until they are cooked through. Serve the soup into bowls.

Break any kind of bread, ideally flatbread, into small pieces and add to the bowl of soup. Mix the bread through for a few seconds until the bread softens slightly.

Serve with fresh herbs like spring onion, radishes, tarragon, and coriander or with fresh onion and homemade pickles.

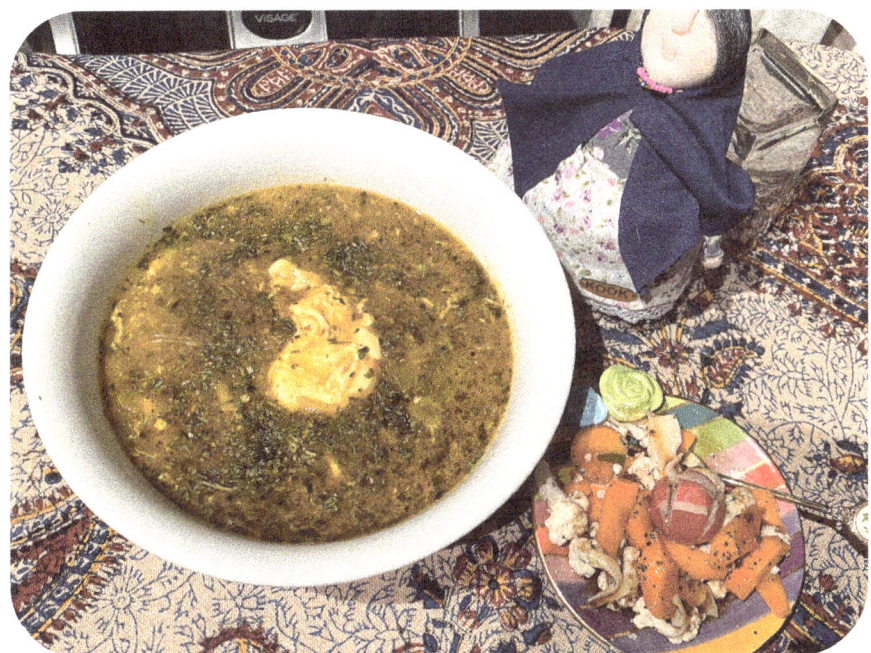

Adasi

Adasi, a slow simmered green lentil soup, is a food with a very long, historic reputation going back nearly 2000 years.

Due to its easy preparation and simple ingredients, it is considered a good food for poor people and one of kids' favourite breakfasts. Adasi means lentil, and is mostly cooked with green lentils, although the same method would work for any other kind of lentils. The best lentils in Iran were grown in the northern part of the very historical province Isfahan.

Although it is mostly served as breakfast, its high nutritional benefits make Adasi useable for lunch or a light dinner too.

Since there was no transportation system, people used to leave the house after morning prayer and before sunrise to be on time for their jobs. Most of the time, they had nothing for breakfast before they left home because it was too early to eat.

People would usually have breakfast in teahouses, but in the streets you could also see men carrying big round pots with trays on top and a few small bowls and spoons. Their pots were full of Adasi.

These men would cook their Adasi the night before to be ready for the next day. After morning prayer, before anyone else left their houses, they would set out with pots of Adasi on their head to seek out their customers. They would sell Adasi in the colder months and in hot seasons, they would sell cold yogurt soup with ice on top as lunch. It was a hard job, since they had to be able to keep their food hot or cold depending on the season, and to sell all of their food before it would lose its desired temperature. Depending on the weather, the vendors would sell their products near their houses so at midday, they could refresh their pots with second batches of their products.

Imagine walking down a snowy street and someone offers you a hot bowl of delicious soup! Adasi was in highest demand in winter, as many believed it was great medicine for cold and flu – especially if cooked with pumpkin. For them, cooked pumpkin in lentil soup was a medicine to soothe their throat and calm down their cough. I have tried it when I had a very bad cough and for some reason it really works, especially when you have it hot …

Although it was often offered as a street food, Adasi was always available as breakfast in teahouses too. Simple, healthy, and above all delicious, Adasi was a reason for many to drop in at a teahouse in the very early morning – even for few minutes – just long enough to eat a bowl to start their day.

Some would come back for lunch but many visits to teahouses were limited to short visits in the early morning and for having a quick breakfast.

Eventually, tea was always served after any kind of breakfast with sugar cubes or Nabat, which is very sweet hard candy. It was and still is believed that Nabat has lots of health benefits. It might seem strange to us that a very sweet candy could have medicinal benefits but Iranians believe it is very useful for your body and your health – especially if you have it with mint tea.

Serves 4

Prep time: 10 minutes

Cooking time: 45 minutes or, for a better result, slow cook on a low heat for longer

- 2 tbsp vegetable oil
- 1 tbsp butter
- 1 medium onion, diced
- 1 medium clove of garlic, finely chopped

- 1 cup dried green lentils
- 3–4 cups stock or water
- 1/2 tsp turmeric
- 1 tsp Angelica powder
- salt and pepper

Method

Add butter to oil in a medium pan.

When the oil is hot, add onion and garlic and fry for 10 to 12 minutes. When the onion and garlic start to turn golden, add the turmeric.

Add lentils and stock or water, and bring to a boil over a high heat.

Once the mixture is boiling, reduce the heat and cover the pan with a lid.

Simmer for 45 minutes, stirring every so often to make sure nothing sticks to the pan, and adding more stock or water if needed. Once lentils are soft, taste to adjust seasoning if needed. When the soup is thick and has absorbed all of the liquid, it's ready. Pour into bowls topped with Angelica powder and more butter if desired. Serve with bread and lemon juice.

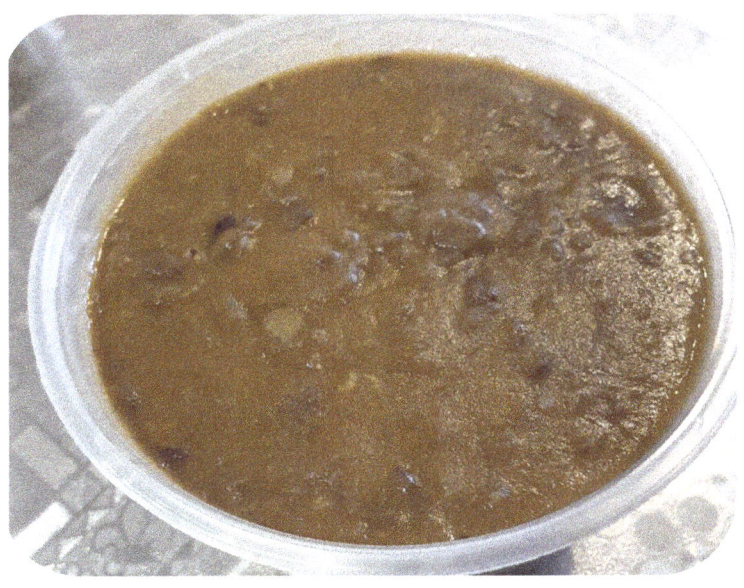

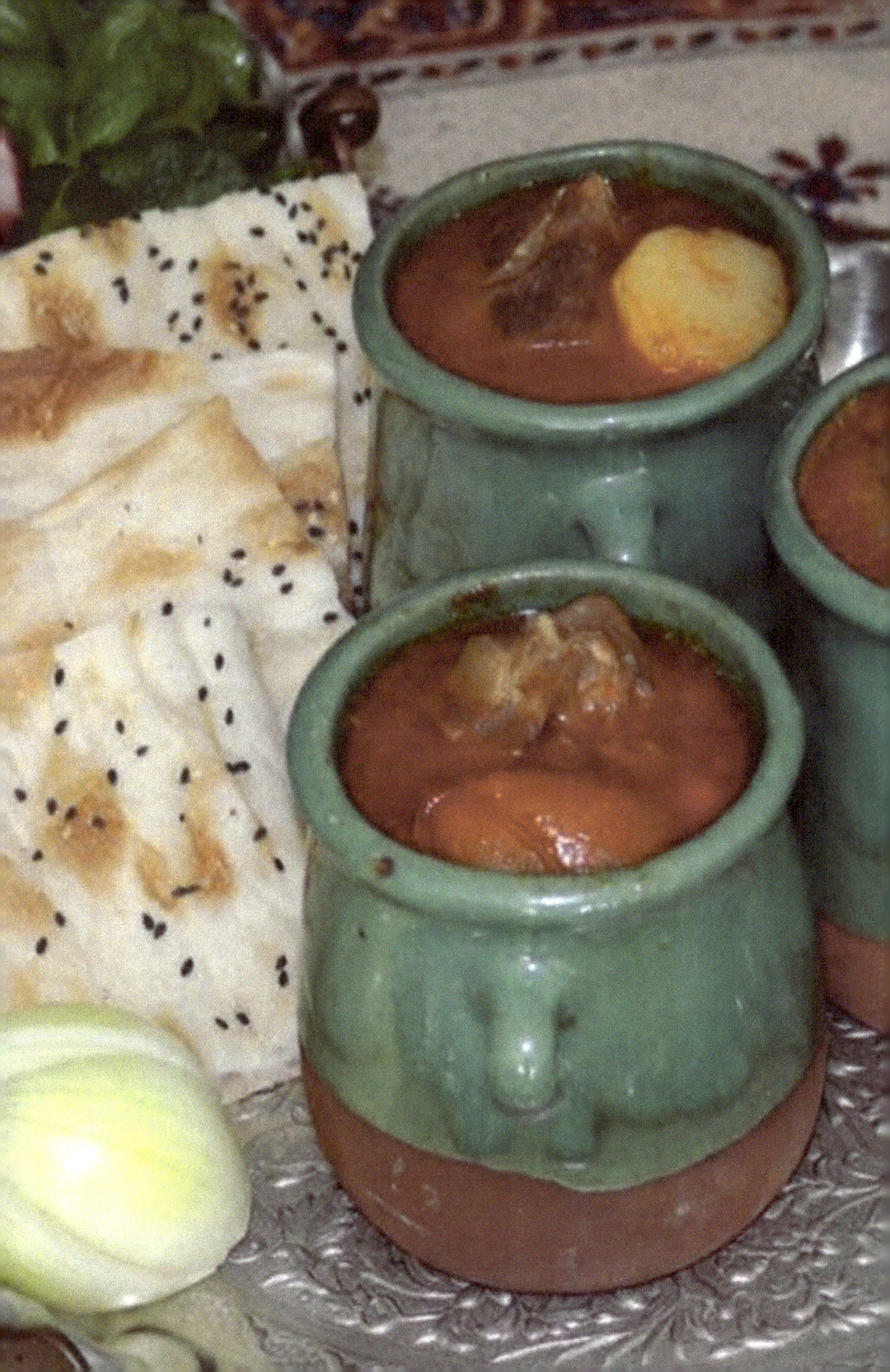

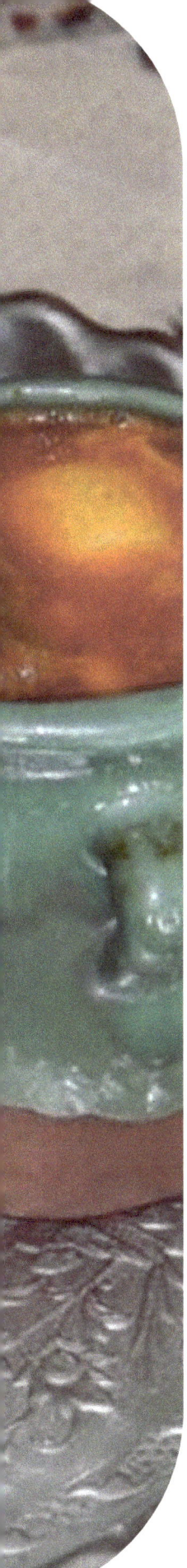

Abgosht

Another common teahouse food is Abgosht, or meat broth. This one-pot comfort food originated as a rustic dish and soon became common all over the country.

The oldest written evidence about Abgosht is in a book of poems by Rumi, dating back to the 13th century. There is a saying that in the old days, people had Abgosht 100 days a year. This might seem like an exaggeration but, like Eshkeneh, the dish originates from a time that men and women mostly used to work together on farms the whole day, not leaving much time for women to practice their daily cooking.

Abgosht is still very popular for busy days today, as you just put all ingredients in one pot and leave it on low heat, preferably overnight, until it's done. Most classic Persian dishes are very time-consuming to prepare but, as they say in Iran, if you're busy with daily tasks, just prepare all the ingredients for Abgosht, leave on a low heat, and go after your life.

While easy to prepare, it's extremely delicious, especially if cooked with fresh and particularly boney lamb, like lamb neck. Although it's quite delicious, it's not normally served to guests and is more of a family dish. If you were to cook it for guests, especially if it's their first time visiting your house, they might get offended. That said, all tourists in Iran have definitely tried it at least once. If you're travelling to Iran for the first time, everybody will recommend you have it, since most teahouses will have it on their lunch menus.

Abgosht is served in a special stoneware crockpot called Dizi, so is sometimes also called Dizi.

It should be eaten in two different steps: first, having the soup or broth in a bowl with broken pieces of bread called Tried, and second when all other ingredients are smashed up, served on a plate and eaten on top of flatbread, with homemade pickles, like garlic pickles, fresh herbs or slices of fresh onion. Traditionally, Abgosht is served with a bread like sangak – a long flat dark bread made with wholemeal flour, baked over hot pieces of stone on a special furnace, rather than an oven.

Serves 4

Cooking time: The best result comes from slow cooking overnight, but the dish could also cook in 3 1/2 hours

- 2 pieces of boney lamb, ideally ribs or lamb shank
- 1 medium onion, quartered
- 1 1/3 tbsp tomato paste
- 1 tsp turmeric
- salt and black pepper
- 2l water
- 1/4 cup white beans, soaked in advance
- 1/4 cup chickpeas soaked in advance
- 2 medium potatoes
- lemon

Method

Set a large soup pot over a high heat and add lamb, onions, tomato paste, turmeric, salt and pepper, and water.

Drain the soaked beans and chickpeas and add to the pot.

Bring to the boil, stirring to dissolve the tomato paste and cover the pot with a lid. Reduce the heat and let it simmer for 3 hours.

After 3 hours, peel and halve potatoes and add to the pot. Continue to simmer for another half an hour, or until the potatoes, meat and beans are all completely tender.

Adjust salt and pepper to taste.

How to eat Abgosht

Use a sieve to remove potato, meat, and beans from the pot and transfer to a large bowl.

Use a potato masher to mash potatoes, meat, and beans to a soft, uniform paste. This paste is called goosht (meat) kobideh (mashed).

If the mixture appears dry, add spoonfuls of broth until smooth but not too soft. Add lemon juice.

For the broth, transfer to a medium bowl and add broken pieces of bread into broth.

Mix and wait until bread starts to soften.

Serve with pickles or fresh herbs.

Then, serve spoonfuls of the goosht kobideh on small broken pieces of flatbread, folded with fresh herbs, or pickles.

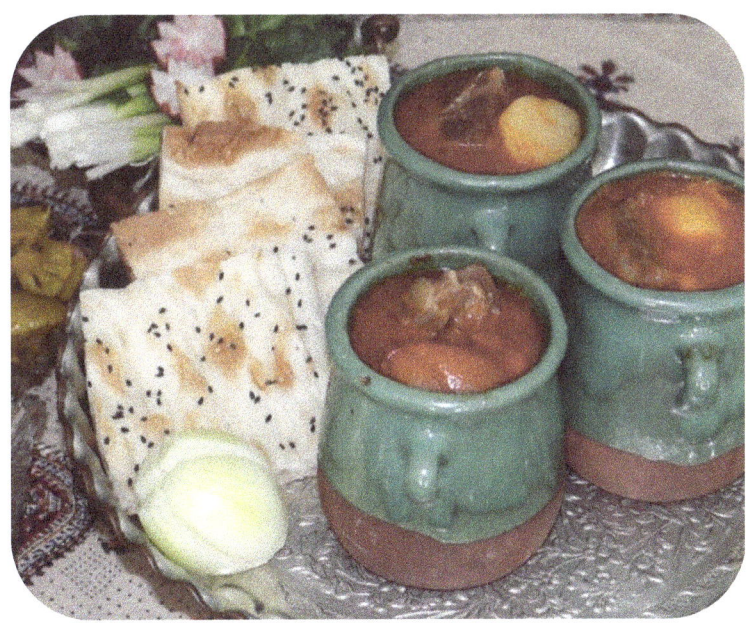

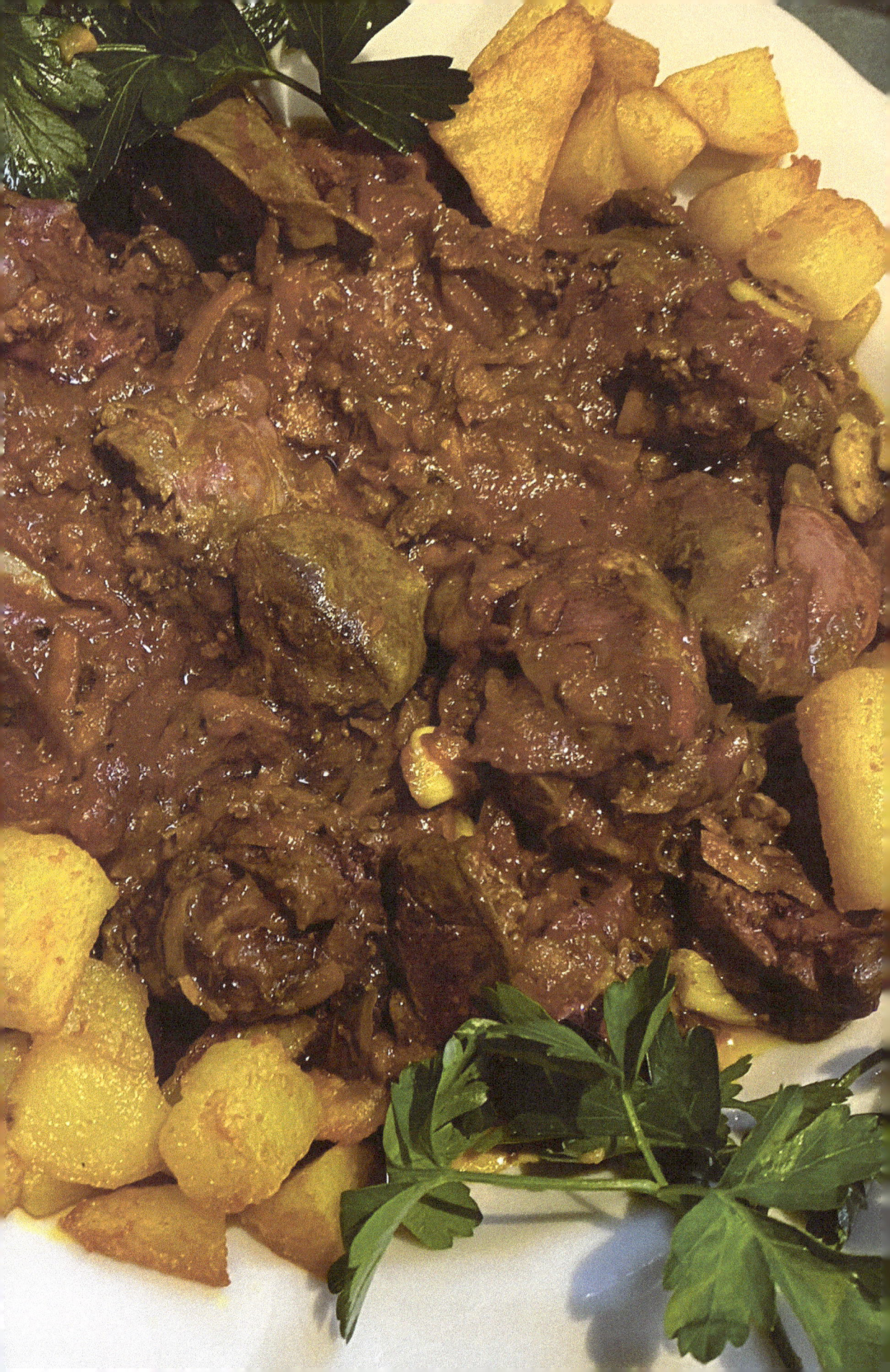

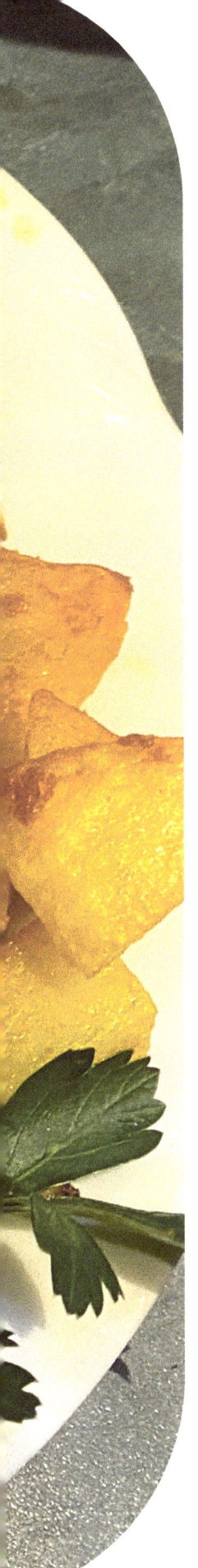

Gaghour Baghour, or Hasrat O Al Molok

In the evenings, people went to teahouses more for entertainment than food. Men tired of daily work would go to leave behind whatever they had experienced during the day – like modern clubs. Most customers would then go home for dinner, so for them this break was only for a short time after work, but some men would have their dinner in a teahouse and stay there till midnight. That made teahouse dinner menus very limited and simple.

One of the most common choices on teahouse dinner menus – sheep liver and heart, either barbecued or cooked on an open flame, mixed with vegetables and spices – was called Gaghour Baghour. This name can even sound strange to Iranian people. It is quick and delicious, so was a very appropriate dish for teahouses.

In some states of Iran it called Hasrat (a wish didn't come true) O Al Molok (a traditional name for women). This second name is taken from an Iranian king's wife. The king and his wife, who was pregnant, were visiting a city called Zanjan. By the time the king's caravan was passing through the streets of Zanjan, someone was cooking Gaghour Baghour. The king's wife asked for the food she could smell (Iranians believe a pregnant woman should eat a bite of whatever she smells otherwise that lack may have an impact on the baby in her womb) but the king's soldiers couldn't find the source of the smell and they had to leave. On their way back to capital, the king's wife felt very sick, and as they got back to the court, she felt even more sick. The court doctors who visited prescribed her to have what she smelled on their journey but hadn't had a chance to eat, so the King sent an ambassador back to Zanjan to ask about the food. They got the recipe and came back to court to ask the court chef to prepare it for the king's wife, Hasrat O Al Molok. As soon as she had it she felt better, so the king also asked to taste it. He liked it so much that he named the food after his wife and that is why this food has two different names in different states. This food is also cooked in Scotland with a different recipe.

Serves 4

Cooking time: 30 minutes

- 1 large onion, sliced
- 500 grams lamb or beef liver, chopped into bite sized pieces
- 1 tbsp high quality turmeric
- 1 tsp salt
- 1 tsp black pepper
- 2 tbsp tomato paste
- 2 medium potatoes, diced
- 8- vegetable oil for frying

Method

Heat vegetable oil in frying pan and fry onion on medium heat until golden.

Add liver and sauté briefly for 3 to 4 minutes.

Once liver has changed colour add turmeric, salt, and pepper and stir briefly. The secret is not to overcook the lamb liver since it only needs a very brief cook to be tender.

Add tomato paste and stir on a low heat for 3 minutes.

Fry potatoes in a separate pan.

Serve warm in the centre of the plate and fried potato around, with fresh herbs and slices of onion.

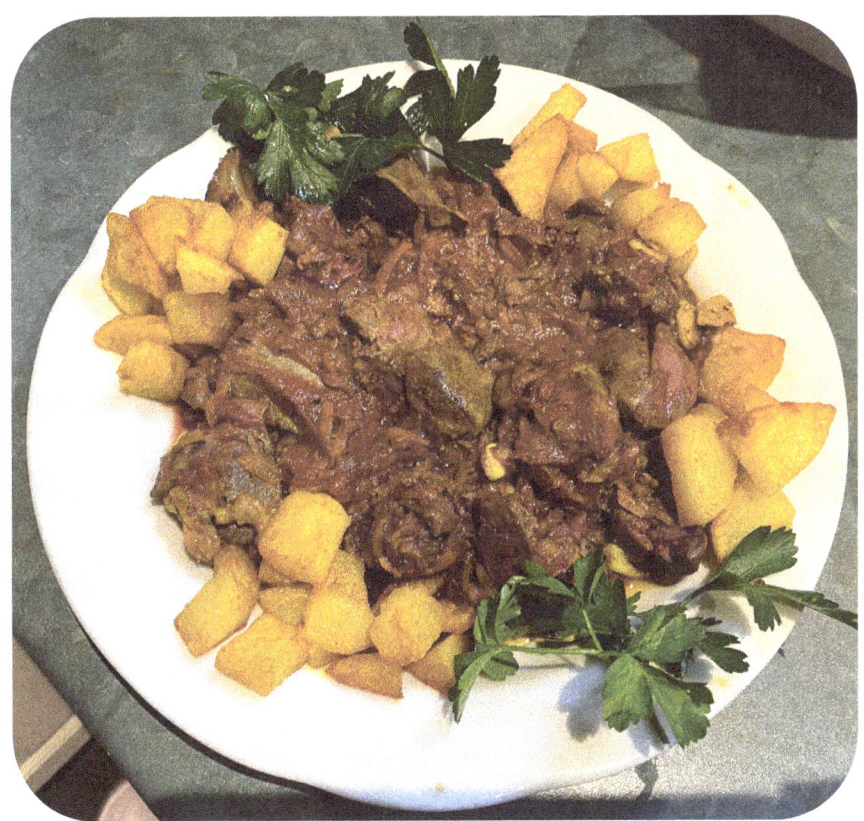

Street food

Street food is one the most popular and favourite styles of food all over the world.

The idea of street food first occurred among labourers who had to work at a distance from their home. Bringing food from home created two problems. Firstly, it was inconvenient, since most of the time they had to walk to work and it was not easy to carry the extra weight. Secondly, in the hot season it was not safe to carry such food since it might perish on the journey.

So, street food started getting popular among poor people and then among others because it was cheap, delicious, fresh, and quick to prepare.

The very first origin of street food can be traced back to ancient Greece, but some say it was in India.

Nowadays, every country has its own street food, although some are common to them all. These foods are also attractive to tourists, not only because of the taste but because of their usually reasonable prices. Besides, it's interesting to eat while you're walking through the streets and looking at people passing by – like you're watching a movie and having your snack at the same time. For those who don't have enough time to sit in restaurants, street food is also an easy option.

In Iran, street food originated in Abadan, in Southern Iran. This was a city with lots of petrol refining factories, so there were large numbers of people from other countries working in this city. These people were not very familiar with local food, and didn't have access to their own local food either, so local workers started sharing their food with them. This made some local workers think they could cook and sell some of these simple foods onsite. This was when street food started getting popular in Iran.

These days, street food is very popular almost everywhere in the country, and each state has their own number one place for street food. What makes these foods so popular is their simple, limited ingredients and fast preparation process which makes them easy to cook in front of customers.

The most famous Iranian street food can be found in the capital city of Tehran, in Si E Tir street.

This is where you can find all sorts of the most popular street foods from all over the country. For someone who is new to Persian street food, and wants to get to know them better, this street in Tehran is probably the best choice.

Almost all the houses along this street are designed in the twentieth century architectural style, and even looking at these buildings from the outside could be fun for a tourist. When I was home, I used to walk down Si E Tir just to look at these buildings from the street. Most of these buildings have their own stories – like a big, spacious building which was the residency of American soldiers and army forces during the Second World War, but is now hired out for socialising purposes by other cultural communities, like Korean and Chinese communities. There are also a few very interesting museums on this street, and it's worth spending a whole day exploring Si E Tir street.

Another famous place to eat street food is Tehran Bazaar, or the famous Tehran market. This was once the most famous marketplace in Iran.

You can find almost everything in this market. All the shops are under roof and on two sides of one aisle. They have the traditional look and reputation of shops from at least two centuries ago, yet in them you can find most modern products, such as the latest technology products.

When you're passing through these aisles, next to almost every shop you will see men (mostly men) with small portable stands selling their street food. Street food is so popular in Tehran Bazaar that there are number of restaurants selling only street food there too. But people visiting the Bazaar mostly prefer to buy street food from stands and traditional food from restaurants.

Some of these restaurants are very famous for particular dishes, and sometimes visitors to the Bazaar will only come to the Bazaar to eat that particular food in one of these famous restaurants. Some of the restaurants in the Bazaar have their own interesting stories too.

The owner of one of the most famous Kabab restaurants, Shamshiri, used to be an assistant in a teahouse, which he later bought, and after a while, turned it into a restaurant with his sister's help. He was also famous because he was advocating for Prime Minister Mosadagh while he was trying for the nationalisation of oil industry. This prime minister had a great impact on

Iranian life as he stood strongly in front of many other countries who were trying to control Iranian policies.

One of the other things that distinguishes these restaurants from other restaurants is the fact that they still have twentieth century furniture, design and dishes and traditional music.

But back to Iranian street food. Vendors used to sell their street food or snacks on wheelbarrows. These were square or rectangular wheelbarrows with a flat surface. Underneath this flat surface, vendors would carry all the equipment and ingredients they needed for cooking.

They would cook their food in front of their customers, as mostly they would prefer to eat the dishes fresh and warm and also to witness the cooking process – this gave them double the pleasure of having street food. That is a bonus you can't get when you're having restaurant food.

Most of the time, street food is offered at much more reasonable prices than restaurant food, which makes it much more affordable for everyone. It also gives people more of a chance to get familiar with their social environment. Perhaps it's always interesting for people to know more about native and local options and food is always the best and most attractive reason to dig in.

Most of the following recipes are taken from popular, well known versions of the food from a particular city, but there are some dishes, such as falafel or finger kabab (small finger-sized minced meat on a skewer with special spices and herbs, fried in oil), that are served in all cities in Iran.

These are the most common and popular Iranian street foods.

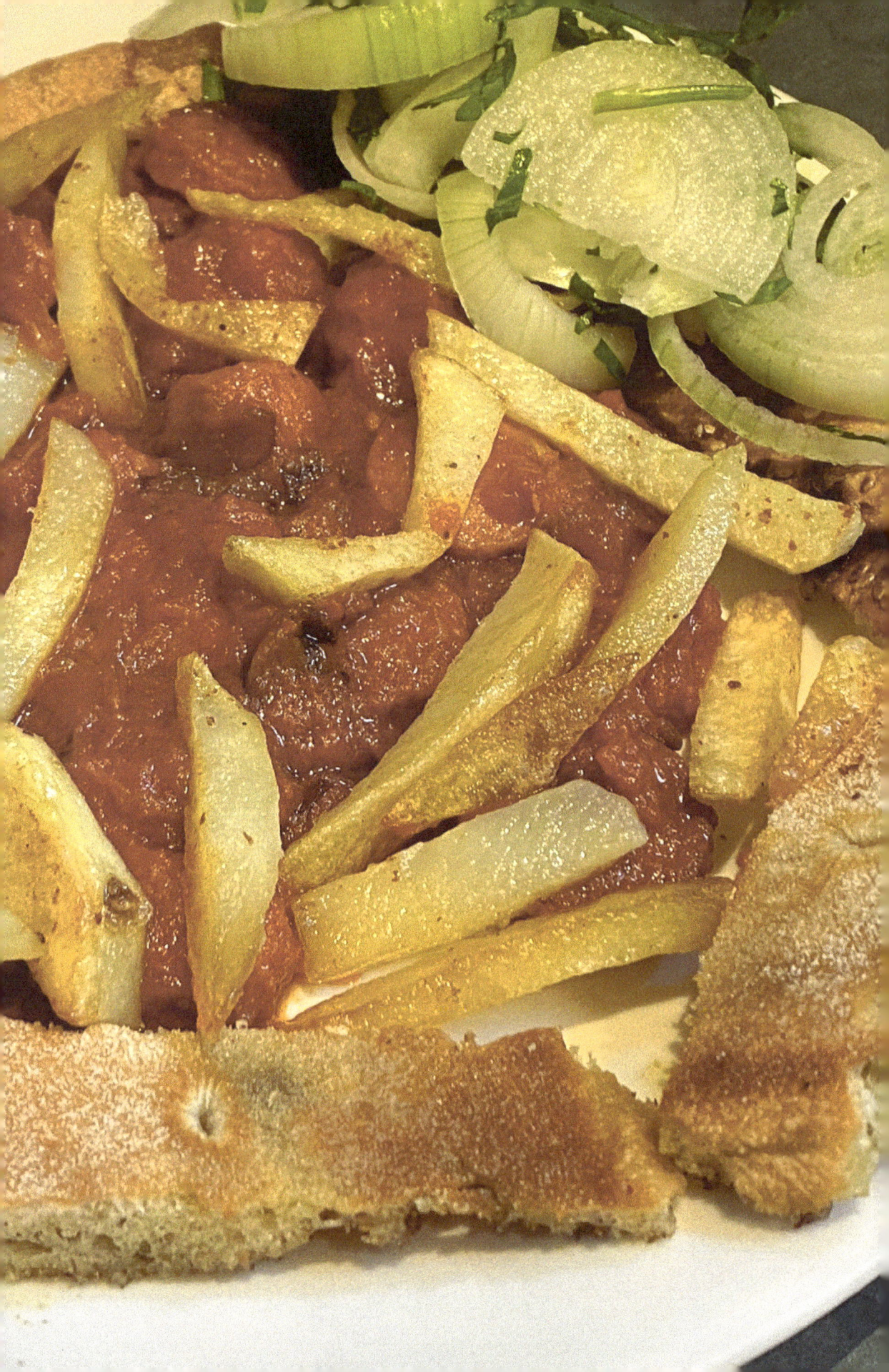

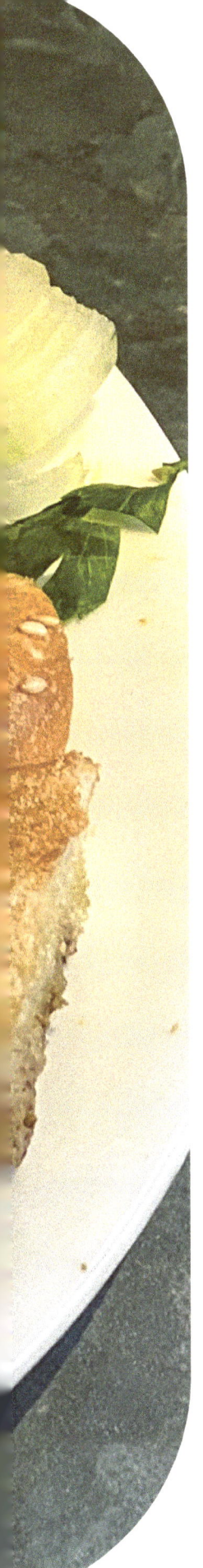

Sosis Bandari

During the Second World War, a number of German, American, and British soldiers were based in different cities of Iran, including Tehran, and some southern coastal cities which were close to ports in the Persian Gulf.

German soldiers who had come from the navy had some of their own cultural food, including some perishable food like sausages, with them. They could use this kind of food in the coastal cities but were not able to take it to other far cities like Tehran. So they had to use these sausages fast before they went off, and they would exchange these sausages with local people for things like cigarettes.

Local Iranian people didn't know how to use these sausages, as Germans usually fried or barbecued them. They also didn't like the taste and couldn't think of these sausages as a meat product: to them, it looked weird. There were rumours that the sausages were made of dogs and pork and – as most locals were Muslim and strictly against dogs and pork – the older generation started banning them. The younger generations didn't mind trying them and invented their own recipes with sausages. Because these recipes were first made in coastal cities, close to the ports, they called this food Sosis Bandari (from a city close to the port): one of the most famous and delicious Iranian street food sandwiches.

Iranians were introduced to sandwiches around the same time. Before, they used to use flatbread – as most Iranian breads are flat – to make a wrap called loghmeh (one piece food).

As the southern states in Iran were close to Arabic countries and they share the same climate, their eating habits are also very much affected by Arabic culture. Here, they eat hot spicy foods which are not very popular in other states in Iran, so this new version of sausage was originally hot too.

Sosis Bandari is simple, fast, but very delicious. Some people have it for breakfast since it's very nutritious and keeps you full for the whole day. It's also one of the most popular birthday party foods as kids love it. I will introduce you to more Persian foods that kids love later in this book.

Serves 4

Prep time: 10 minutes

Cooking time: 20 minutes

- 3 medium potatoes, peeled and diced
- 500g sausages, sliced
- 1/3 cup vegetable oil, for frying
- 3 medium onions, sliced
- 3 tbsp tomato paste
- 1 tsp turmeric
- ½ tsp hot chilli (optional)
- ½ tbsp curry powder (optional if you like it hotter)
- salt and black pepper

Method

Fry the potatoes in vegetable oil and set them aside.

Then, fry the sausages in 2 tablespoons of the vegetable oil and set them aside.

Fry the onion in the oil until moderately caramelised.

Add turmeric, curry powder, and tomato paste to the caramelised onion. Then add 1/4 cup of water and the sausages and stir on low heat until the sauce starts getting thick.

Remove from the heat, dish up and top with the fried potato.

If you like it as sandwiches, serve the mixture into fresh bread rolls with lettuce leaves.

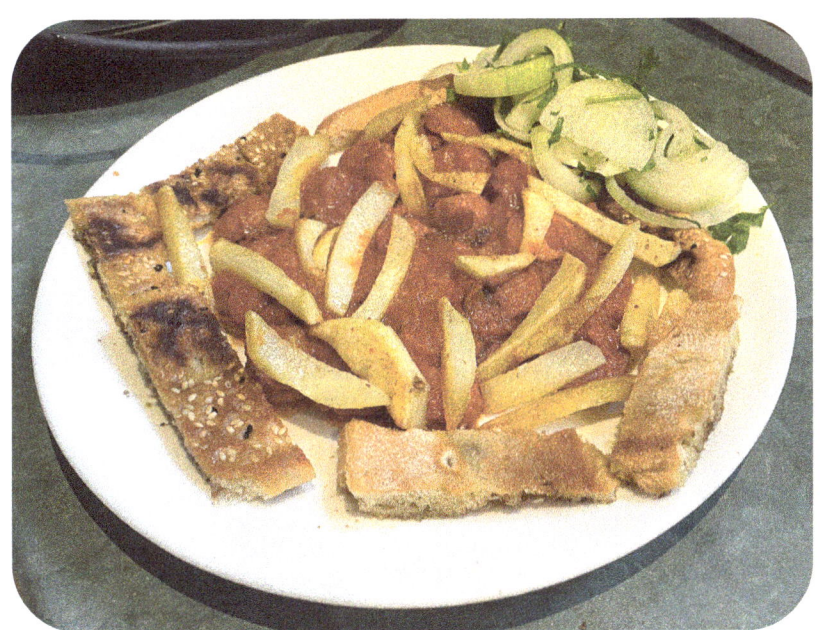

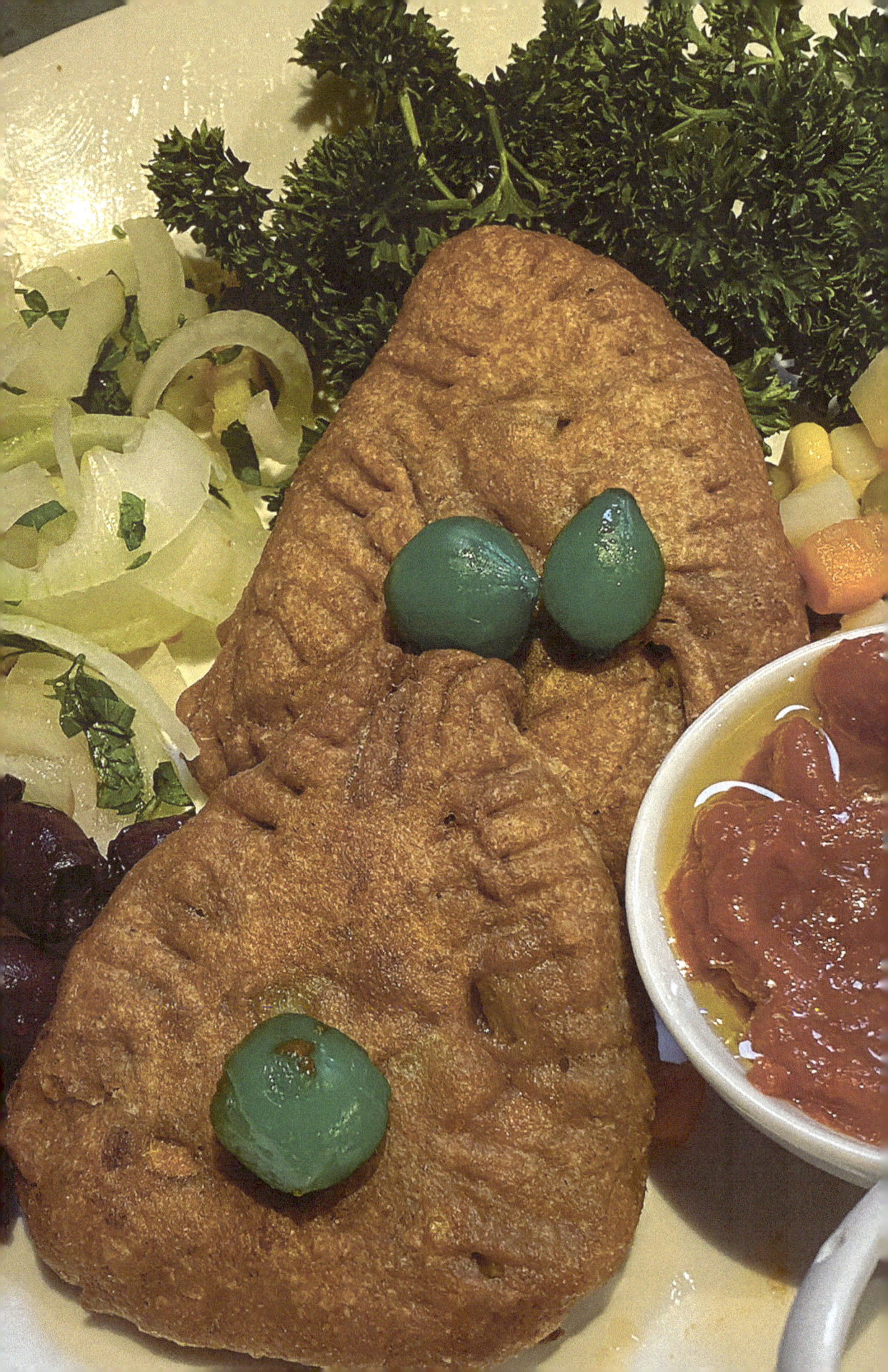

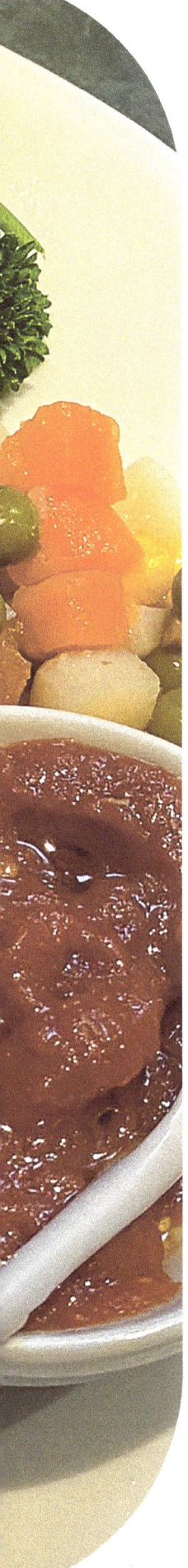

Samosa

Samosas are a very well known snack all around the world. People believe the origin of samosas is India, but the very first version of them originated in northeastern Iran in the Khorasan province, as is written in Abou Fazel Beyhaghi's book from the 11th century.

The first version of these delicious little triangles was actually not what we enjoy as a snack but one of the ingredients in a special kind of soup eaten by residents of northeastern Persia.

People all over the country started to know this delicious soup and its tasty, little, floating triangles and it became very popular. It was later used by the Ghaznavi empire's noble people of the court.

Today it is one of the most famous street foods, not only in Persia and India, but all around the world, and you can hardly find anyone who hasn't tried it

Despite the fame these little delicious triangles carry, it is probably hard to believe that nearly 50 years ago, only residents of southern states in Iran had tasted it and knew it as a street food.

Samosas and falafel were unknown or forgotten street food for people from other states in Iran because people from the late '50s and early '60s started knowing more about western style street food in Iran.

However, in the late '80s Iranian people started getting more familiar with other states' local food. This was beause during the early revolution years and the start of sanctions, it was not easy to have access to lots of ingredients and recipes from a broad range of countries.

People who live in the southern states of Iran have saved it in their daily menu for thousands of years and have been so loyal to their traditional recipes. Thanks to this loyalty, we have lots of amazing recipes from different states all over the country.

Today if you walk in the cities of the southern states' you can see street food vans selling these two foods all over the cities. Some only sell these two and that proves these two snacks have a very special place in their daily food menu.

The original version of samosa was nothing like what we have today. It was first limited to a dough prepared from wheat, water, and salt which is well-kneaded and filled with cooked, smashed chickpeas, fried onion, minced meat, and spices like turmeric, black pepper and local spices, wrapped into small triangle shapes and boiled in the broth of a soup called Joush Pareh (Joush = boiling). Later, it was called Sambusak or Sambosang soup (triangle soup, as in the local language Sambosang = triangle).

When Indian merchants travelled to the northeastern states they loved the food, but it seemed they were more interested in the little triangles floating in the broth rather than whole soup. When they took the recipe to their homeland, they changed it to what we call samosas today. By skipping the broth and boiling process, only the dough and its filling continued to be used, as it was their main interest.

They also changed the boiling process to deep frying for the dough. Of course, frying made a more delicious version of it and soon everyone fell in love with this new version of samosas. The filling was also changed according to their traditional desired taste which tends to be a lot more hot and spicy.

This new version of samosa was later transferred back to the southern states of Iran by Iranian merchants from southern Iran, who travelled to India to import fabrics to Iran as the variety and quality of fabrics in India was and still is very famous among all merchants.

They tasted this new version and found it more interesting and more tasty. Finally its specifications, shape, and cooking process changed to what we have today for samosa.

Southern states were so close to Arabic counties and both areas are very much affected by each other's culture, traditions, and of course food. This new version of samosas was introduced to Arabic countries and became one of the first choices on their street food menu and for a daily snack.

If you go to any street food shop in the southern states of Iran, you will find a huge range of different kinds of samosa in their menu with versatility in fillings and lots of different tastes.

Usually the ingredients for dough are the same in all sorts of samosas, though in some cases there are slight changes in ingredients and process of dough making. However, for the filling they enjoy using a wide range of ingredients and flavours and a wide range of homemade sauces. The combination of all these together amaze all the customers and visitors at these street food shops.

Although you can enjoy the same variety of samosas in street food shops all over the country today, enjoying a delicious samosa was only possible in the southern states of Iran only 50 years ago.

Whether it's cooked for any kind of celebration or for daily use, a decent samosa must be crispy and flaky. Hearing and feeling that crunch proves that the samosa is what it should be.

Although the dough can be wrapped in any shape, a samosa is best in triangular shape. Any other shape rather than triangles doesn't affect the taste, but samosas are mostly known for their triangle shape as best feature.

Vegetarian samosas are more common rather other versions, however, there are no limitations for using any kind of meat in the filling too.

Serves: 4

Prep time: 50 minutes (dough and filling and frying in total)

Cooking: 10 min for each piece

Filling

Here I'm going to give you the recipe for a vegetarian samosa.

Although as I said earlier that samosa is very versatile in filling and of course in taste, the most common one is the vegetarian samosa, in which potato is usually the hero ingredient along with crispy, golden, fried onion flakes, tumeric, paprika, salt, and pepper.

For extra flavour, some add some fried garlic flakes too. I think adding garlic enhances the flavour but it's optional.

Very well chopped parsley also adds more taste to every bite.

The best filling comes from a perfect balance of flavour and texture.

Boiled and grated potato shouldn't be too mushy or chunky and the filling should be aromatic with the spices used.

Of course it's not as hot and spicy as an Indian version but the spices used in the filling still have a major role in the taste of every samosa.

For filling:

(for filling of 4 medium sized samosas)

- 1 large boiled potato, peeled and grated
- 1 medium sized onion, well chopped and fried
- 1/2 tsp tumeric
- 1/4 tsp paprika
- 1/4 tsp chillies
- 2 tbsp fresh parsley, well chopped
- 1/4 tsp black pepper
- salt, as desired

Method

Combine all ingredients in a bowl and set aside to prepare dough.

Dough

To be honest, for an easier process I recommend using ready-made pastry from the market but if you are looking for some dough making here are the steps:

- 2 cup of refined flour
- 1/2 tbsp of salt
- 2 cups of cold water
- 2 tbsp of oil

Method

1. In a large bowl add the salt and flour and rub the oil into it.

2. Add water and knead in to a stiff dough. Stiff dough is very important in this stage (when ready rest for 15 minutes or so)

3. Shape dough in small balls, continue on kneading and cut each ball in to halves

4. Take one half, wet the edge, fold the straight edge at the centre and join by one half overlapping the other to form in to a cone triangle shape

5. Press the overlapping portion and fill with the desired filling (our filling here is enough for 4 medium size samosa. You can prepare other versions of filling to be used for left over dough and try different versions of it, the good thing about this dough is if covered and kept in fridge it can be used later again)

6. Leave frying oil on the medium heat and let it be hot enough to fry Samosa. The oil temperature is very important, it must have enough heat to get best golden colour out of the dough and will give you a great samosa crunch .

Leave each one in the hot oil then lower down the heat and let it go crispy and crunchy.

When you see that golden colour in your samosa take it out with a spatula and leave each on kitchen paper towel to take away that extra oil.

There is also another frying process which is best for people who care about health awareness issues.

Brush the dough with oil on every edge and leave in oven for 7 minutes for each side. Ideally served with fresh herbs or pickles but your free to serve with any kind of sauce you like.

My favourite homemade sauce is with:

- 1 table spoon of mango powder
- 1/4 table spoon of djion mustard
- 1/4 table spoon of pomegranate molasses
- 1/4 grated onion
- 1 grated glove of garlic

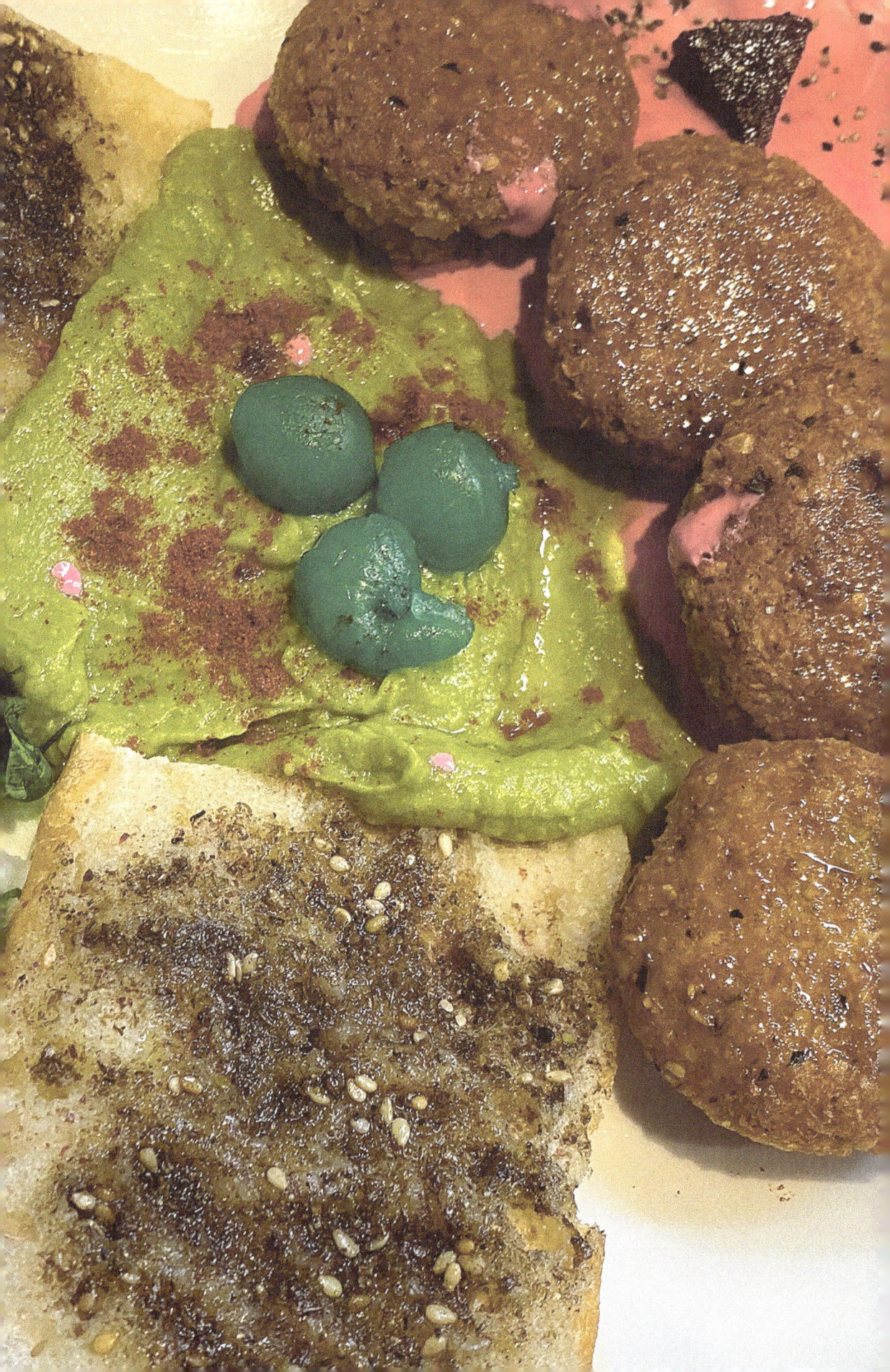

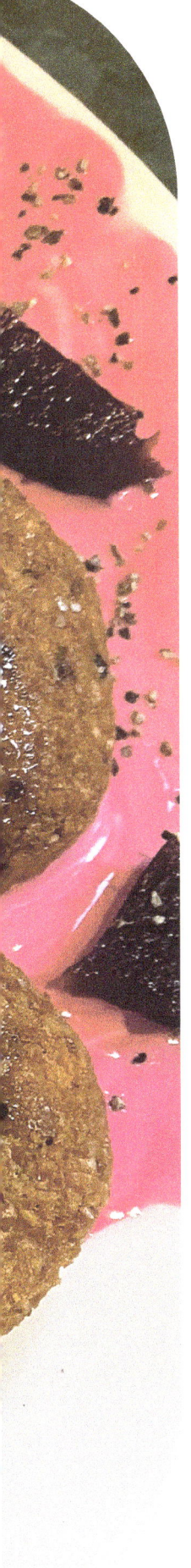

Falafel

Falafel has travelled a long way to our table – it passed through many Arabic countries before it was introduced to the Iranian street food menu.

Invented by Christian Egyptians fasting from meat products on certain days of each month, falafel was not only delicious but cost effective too, and it quickly became popular.

Except for the southern cities in Iran, no one in Iran knew anything about falafel until about 30 years ago, when it was introduced from Iraq after the war between in Iran and Iraq in 1981. This was a turning point in its popularity. It was then that falafel became common among different states.

Nowadays, not only is falafel one of the most famous street foods in Iran, it is also considered a very healthy, nutritious dish among Iranians – even sold in schools.

Falafel is plural for a single word (felfel = chilli) as this is a food with a hot taste. But the Iranian version of falafel is less spicy than the Arabic recipe (as Iranians are not big fans of very hot food, except in the southern cities close to the Arabic countries).

Falafel is usually served with different sides. As you step into a falafel shop in Tehran, you will see a huge range of options, but the most common are special vegetable pickles, mango sauce, hot tomato sauce or simply fresh herbs.

Falafel is also one of the cheapest sandwiches you could have these days. Its affordable price is another element in its growing popularity, as the economic crisis in Iran has changed people's eating habits and maybe their taste as well.

Serves 4

Prep time: 2 hours

Cooking time: 30 minutes

- 1 kg chickpeas, soaked in cold water overnight (change water every 6–7 hours)
- 5 cloves garlic
- 1 medium onion.
- 2 tsp cumin powder
- 1 tsp coriander powder
- Chilli powder (to taste)
- 1 tbsp chickpea flour
- Salt and black pepper
- Vegetable oil, for frying

Method

Blend chickpeas in a food processor to a very smooth paste. Add garlic and onion and continue to blend.

Transfer the paste to a bowl and add the remainder of the ingredients. Mix well and leave it in cold place for two hours.

After two hours, make small balls from the dough, giving each ball a little pressure to make it look like a thick coin. Apply enough pressure to make sure there are no cracks on any of the sides. Wet your hands once a while to make this process easier.

Heat oil to a boil in a small deep pan, then drop falafels in the oil. Fry them in batches for three minutes, or until golden.

Remove the falafels onto paper towel to soak up any excess oil.

Serve on a plate or in flatbread with salad, fresh herbs and pickles and ideally, mango hot sauce (which you can buy from Indian or Persian shops) or but any other kind of sauce.

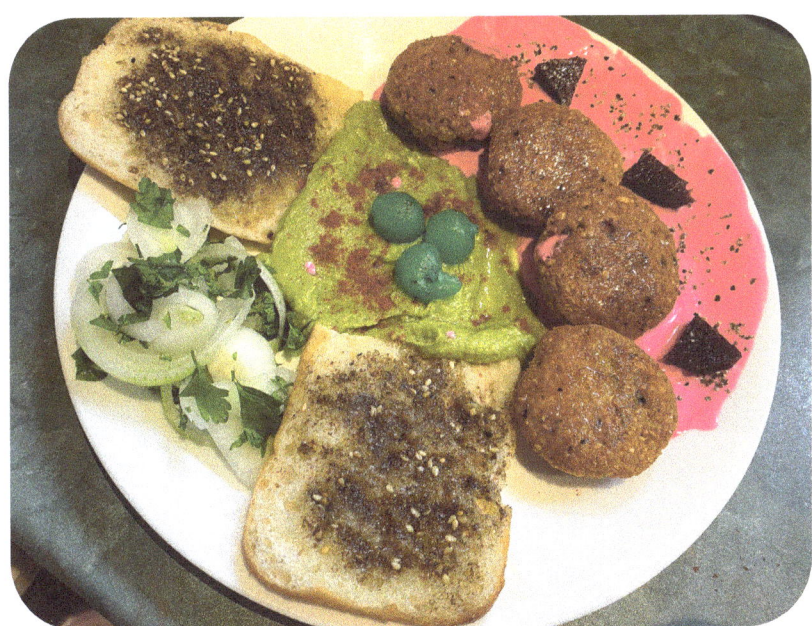

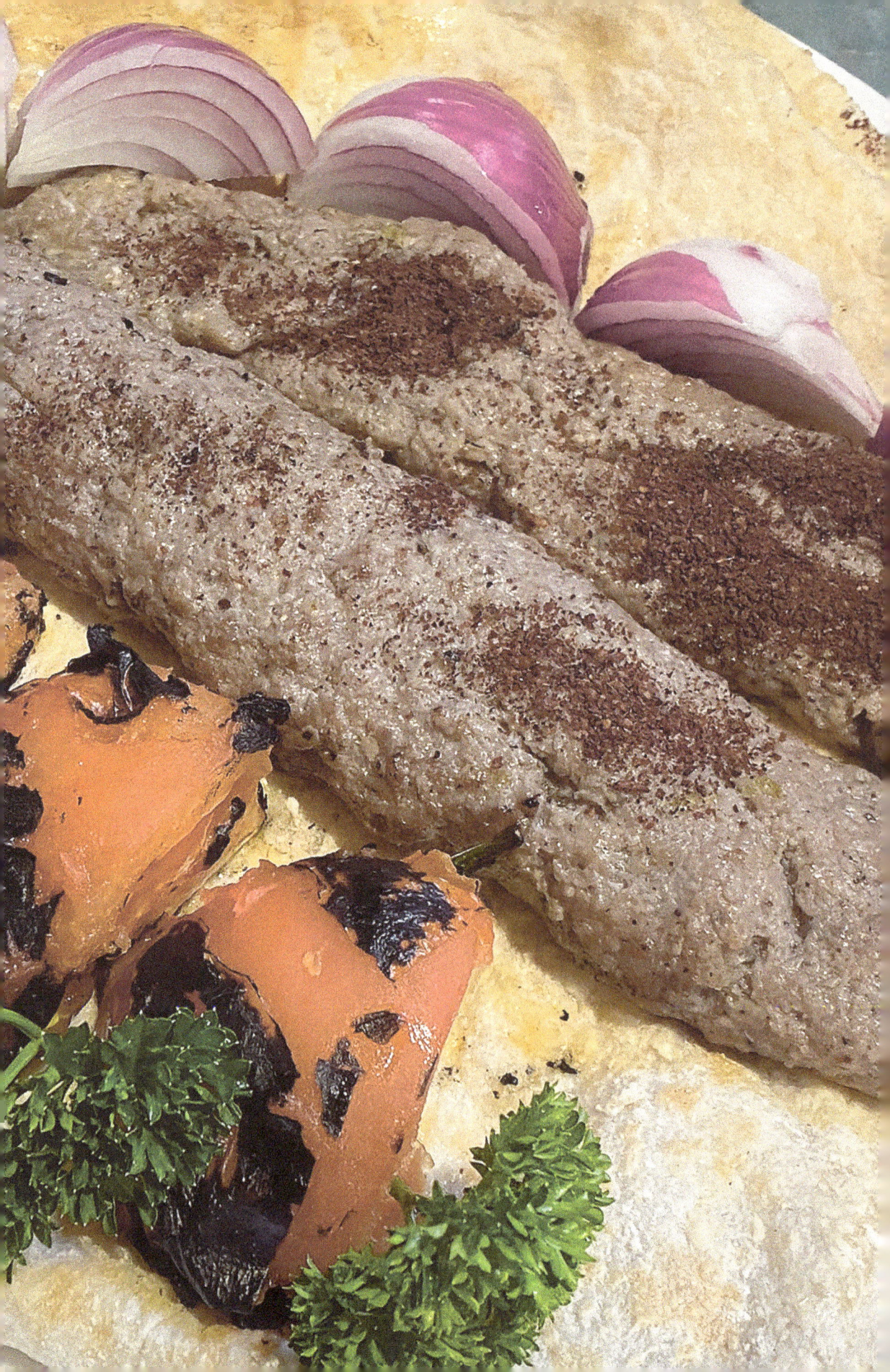

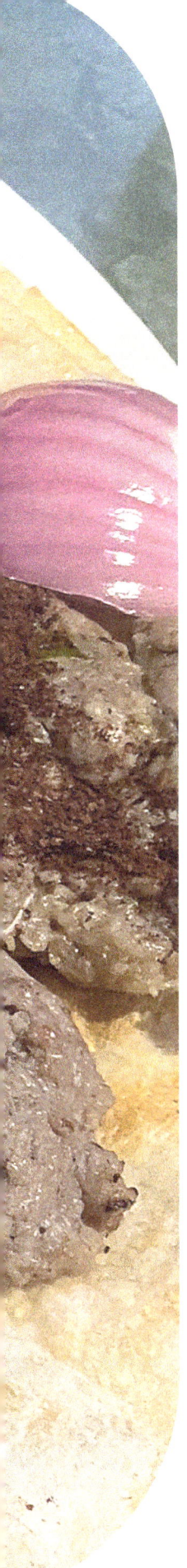

Kabab Loghmeh

Loghmeh means to 'savour in one bite' and as you may know, kabab means barbecue meat over flame. There are variety of kabab in Iran.

Kabab originated from street food, but Iranians love kabab so much, you can find it in almost every restaurant in the country. While there are still street versions of Kabab Loghmeh, and they are fairly delicious, these days, kabab is considered to be one of the most luxurious restaurant foods.

Kabab is originally from Caucasus. During the Qajar dynasty, the king was from the province of Tabriz, close to Caucasus. Since they shared borders, people from these two regions exchanged a lot – including food. So when the king came to the capital city to start ruling, he ordered the court chef to cook kabab. In the only cookbook left from that time, written by court chef, kabab is also called Kabab looleh (tube) since the finished product looks like a tube.

Soon, ordinary people found out about kabab, and among them there was a man selling street food. He started cooking kabab with minced meat in small pieces as small bites so people could afford it. For people in better financial situations, he made bigger ones, on thick skewers, but shaped each piece so it could be torn easily into parts like a small bite for each person. This shop was called Nayeb, and is still a restaurant in Iran, selling different kinds of kabab, called Nayeb. This is where you can find some of the most luxurious, expensive best quality kabab in Iran

Soon, all the other states in Iran were attracted to this interesting food, and each one followed the original recipe but added their own city's flavour. These days, although there are many different recipes for Kabab Loghmeh, the original recipe forms the base part to start the process.

Kabab Loghmeh is also called Kabab Koobideh – since there were no electric meat grinder in the old days to mince the meat – people used to smash the meat in a big mortar and pestle. This smashing was called Koobideh.

To cook Kabab Loghmeh, you will need charcoal and special wide skewers. Ideally, Kabab Loghmeh uses a 2:1 ratio of lamb to beef, since lamb is more fatty. Some think this is the tastiest Kabab since it's fatty and soft. Melting fat over charcoal – or as the expression goes, the kabab's tears – brings up a very delicious smell that makes you feel hungry no matter how full you are.

When it's cooked, kabab is placed on flatbread with a good pinch of sumac and thick slices of onion, then covered with the other layer of flatbread to pull and separate Kabab from skewers. This should be done very fast – first, to keep the kabab warm and second, so the kabab holds its shape and doesn't fall apart. If it breaks, it's still very tasty, but keeping the shape is considered an important element of a good kabab.

The best sides for kabab are barbecued whole tomatoes, fresh onion and basil, served on freshly baked Sangak (long flat dark bread made with wholemeal flour). To attract more customers, some restaurants bake Sangak in an old fashioned furnace on site.

Serves 4

Prep time: 1 hour

Cooking time: 30 min

- 400 grams lamb mince with fat (ideally rib meat)
- 150 grams beef mince
- 2 medium onion, grated and drained well (it very important to drain grated onion otherwise meat won't stick to the skewers)
- Salt and black pepper

- 1/2 tbsp flour
- 1 tsp saffron, brewed with either ice or boiling water (not both)
- 1/2 tsp turmeric
- 6 tomatoes, washed and scored in a cross at the top
- ½ tbsp sumac, plus extra for serving
- 50 grams butter, melted

Method

Flatbread

Skewers (for street food style kabab use small skewers; for restaurant style, use large wide skewers)

Charcoal, if possible (getting the right temperature and flame on charcoal is very important)

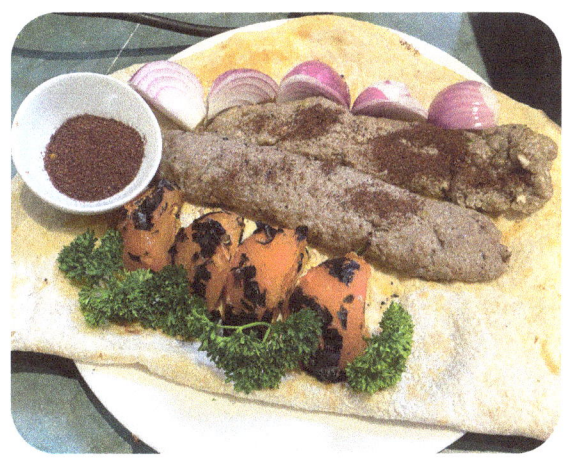

Mix minced meat, onion, salt and pepper, flour, saffron and turmeric well. Add sumac to taste (for kabab, sumac is optional, and used like salt to enhance the taste). Set aside in the fridge for at least 30 minutes.

Skewers the tomatoes on and place over the flame. Once the skin starts to break and the tomatoes are almost soft, take them off the heat and leave on the flatbread. Keep in a warm place until ready to serve with kabab.

Portion the kabab mix into balls roughly the size of a mandarin and put on skewers, making sure the mix is spread evenly over the skewers on all sides. Brush gently with melted butter.

Put the skewers over a medium heat, turning every now and then so the kabab cooks evenly on all sides.

If you don't have access to charcoal or a proper barbecue, fry the kabab in oil or bake in oven at 180 degrees for 15 minutes, remembering to turn skewers every few minutes.

Remove skewers from the heat, take the skewers out slightly and leave on flatbread, topping with the rest of the sumac. Serve with barbecued tomatoes, fresh basil and fresh chunks of onion with flatbread.

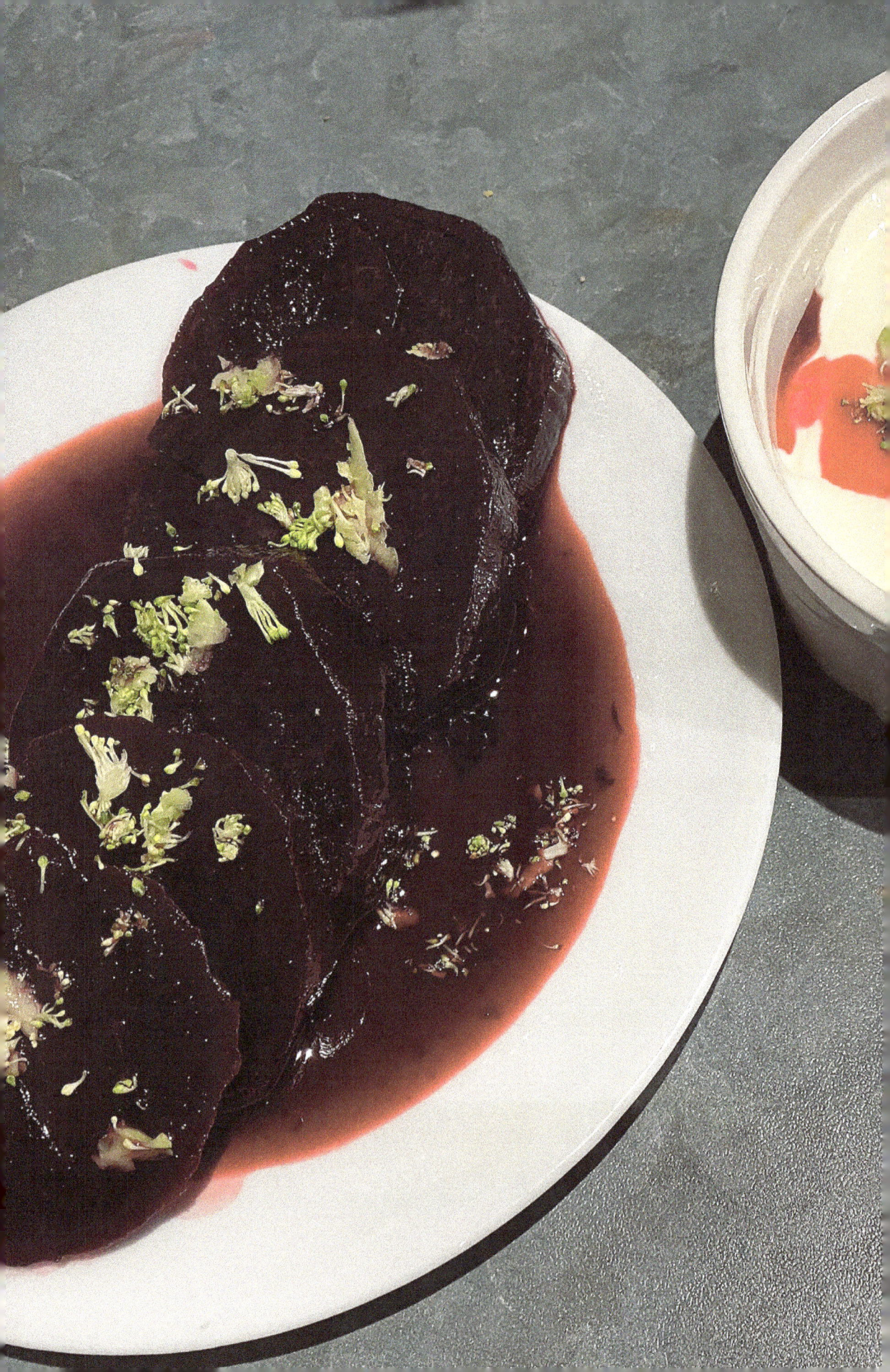

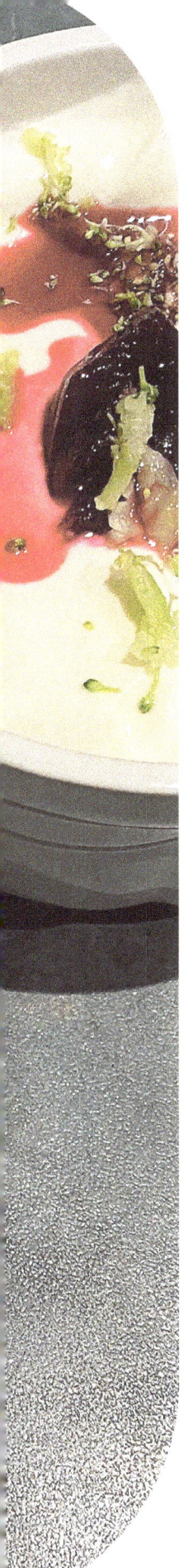

Laboo
(hot beetroots in syrup)

If you ever travel to Iran in winter, there is a familiar scene of wooden, square open caravans carting hot cooked beetroot (laboo) or bread beans (baghali) to sell in the streets. On a cold winter's day, what could be more pleasant than a snack of hot cooked red beetroot or broad beans with touch of dried Angelica or thyme with salt and vinegar?

Whether you're interested in buying these foods or not, there is much beauty in these traditions: the open wooden caravan which looks like a dining table with its warming system underneath, the light from a big oil lamp, the way vendors sing to customers to persuade them to buy their foods, and the colour and scent of these foods. Sellers usually have special, very rhythmic songs that they sing for each one of these products to introduce you to what they are selling. Since it's winter and the food is supposed to be offered very hot, they sing: 'Run Run it's hot (laboo) or (baghali)'. Sometimes, sellers might add a few more words to their song.

Buyers will usually stand around the caravans and eat the food there and then while it's still hot, talking each other or just watching others passing by. All the while, the vendor is still singing to attract more customers.

Sometimes in winter, when there is a lot of cold and flu around, having hot cooked beetroot is a classic Iranian grandma's prescription. Whether it works for your cold or not still doesn't take away from the delicious taste on a very cold day – especially on snowy days when people walk fast through the streets. It's very interesting to stand around one of these warm, wooden caravans – almost like being next to a fireplace – watching people pass by as you eat your hot Laboo.

Serves 4

Cook time: 4 to 5 hours

- 2 big red beetroots, washed and brushed (skin on)
- 3 tbsp sugar
- 5 glasses (1.25 L) water

Method

Boil beetroots over a low heat for four hours to let them cook gradually. Add more water if needed.

After four hours or so, use a fork to check if beetroots are cooked. If the fork gets through easily, the beetroots are cooked. If not, continue cooking, adding more water to pot.

Once cooked, take the pot off the heat and let the beetroots cool down in the liquid (at least two glasses of water should be left in the pot).

Once cool, peel the beetroots and cut into big chunks.

Return the beetroots to the pot. Add sugar and cook for on low heat again for one more hour.

The dish is ready when the water is reduced to half a glass. Turn off the heat. A thick syrup should be left in the pot.

Dish up the cooked beetroots on a plate, pouring the syrup on top. Serve straight away.

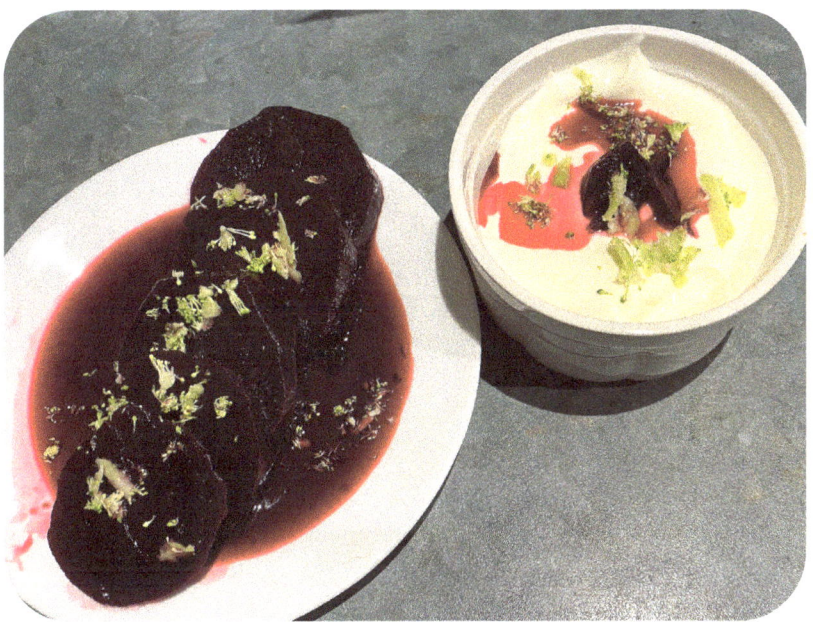

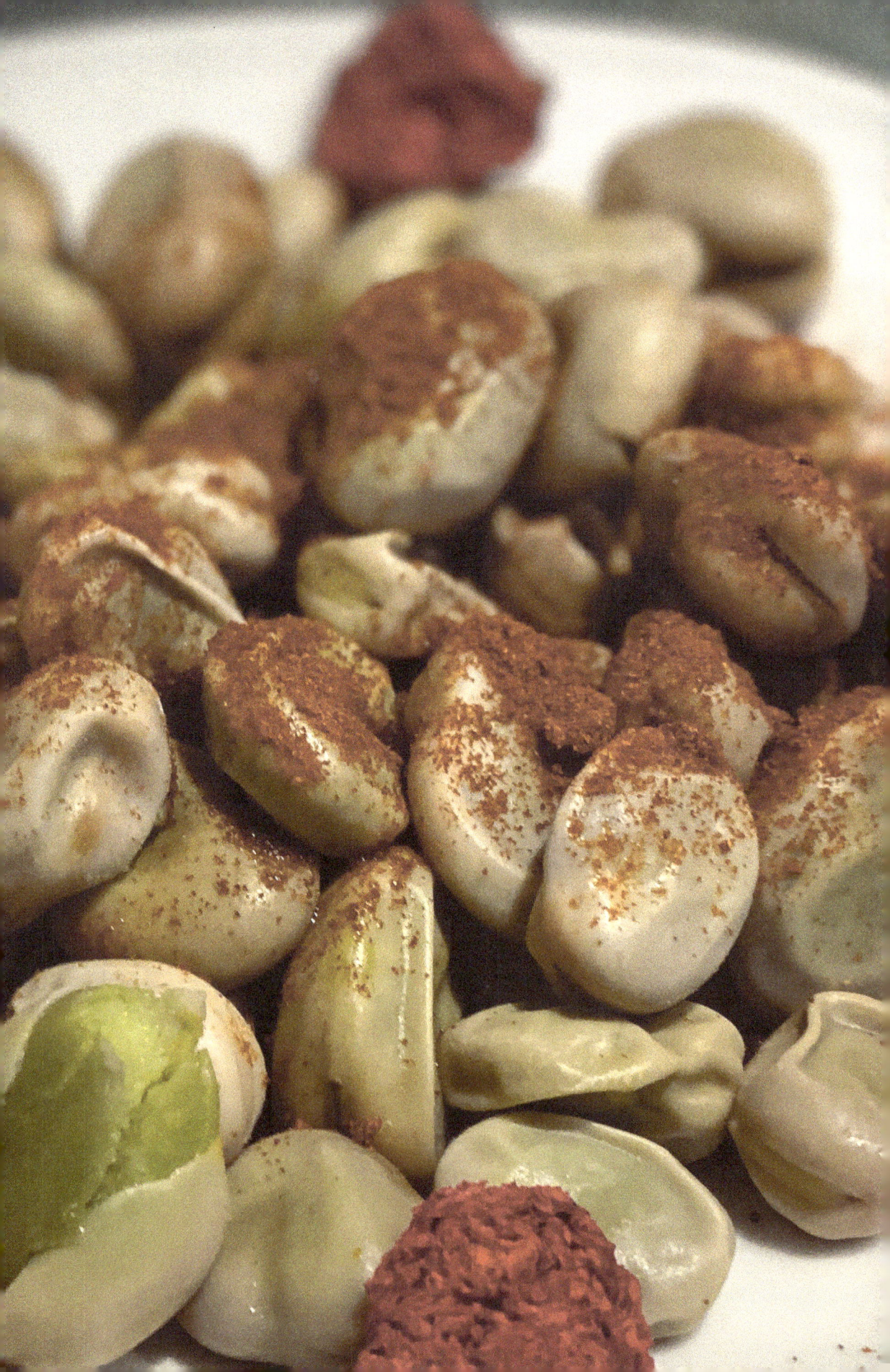

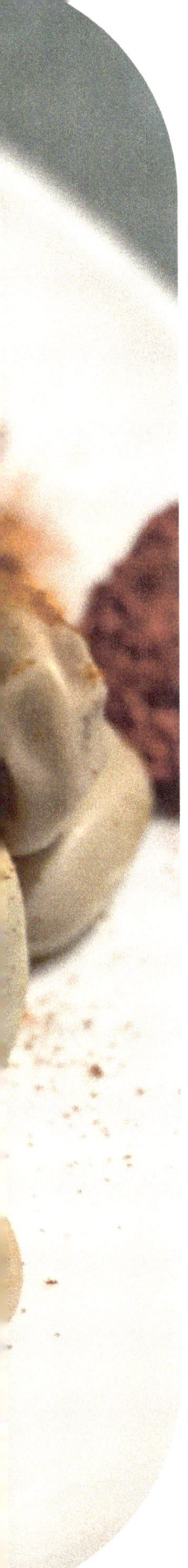

Baghali
(hot broad beans)

Everything in Tehran, the capital of Iran has a story – even a lot of Iranians don't know some of these stories. Through modern, mechanised living we have learned to follow our daily routines and habits – including our eating style – with no thought to the stories behind these habits. But not only are these stories interesting, carrying deep descriptions of culture, they also teach us a lot about how to improve our daily routines and reach our goals and dreams in easier and less stressed ways.

When we follow our lifestyle without thinking, we just know we are not feeling good as we did in our childhoods, and we don't think about why. But one of the reasons we are not feeling good is because we are not paying attention to the stories behind everything. We used to ask about these stories and dig into them to discover life, to build our minds and fulfil our souls. By the time it came to sleep, we used to listen to these beautiful stories to sculpture and engineer our dreams, instead of thinking about our problems and even turn our dreams into nightmares.

Hot beetroot and broad beans are mostly offered in Tehran, where they originated.

Selling broad beans might be a little harder than selling beetroots since they are sold out of season, in winter. So sellers buy them fresh in spring and dry them. They are shelled from their pod, and dried in their skins. These street vendors are usually from a poorer class in society, and live in small houses where they dry and save large amount of broad beans. Otherwise, selling cooked broad beans is almost same process with cooked beetroot.

Usually, vendors sell beetroots in the morning and broad beans in afternoon or both at the same time – Half and half on their cart. People passing by have a hard time deciding which one they should try, hardly anyone chooses both at the same time: first, because they don't think the mixture of the taste would be pleasant, and second because these two foods are both considered to be cold in nature (Iranian people divide the nature of food to hot in nature or cold in nature). This traditional medical belief says that if you have too many hot (in nature) or too many cold (in nature) foods, that would affect your health. So, they usually try to bring a balance between hot and cold: if they have a hot (in nature) food they have something cold (in nature) afterwards to give their body a balance.

The recipe for this street snack will depend on if you're cooking it in or out of season. It's usually something people will have in the early afternoon or early evening before dinner – never after dinner since they believe it's hard to digest and can give them an upset tummy.

If using fresh broad beans

Simply wash broad beans, and leaving them in their pods, cover with water in a big pot and bring to the boil. Add salt as you desire. Once soft, remove from the heat and drain.

Dish broad beans up. Mix salt, Angelica powder and vinegar and pour on top, making sure the sauce covers all parts of the broad beans. In this version, using fresh broad beans, even the outer pod could be eaten, but do not eat too many as they're hard to digest.

Remove the beans from their skin. If they're cooked well, they should come out easily. Mix well with sauce and eat them while still hot.

If using dried broad beans

Serves 4

Cooking time: 3 hours on low heat.

- 200 grams dried broad beans (you can either dry them in their skins in the sun, having removed them from their pods, or buy them from any Persian shops around), soaked in cold water overnight (change water every 6–7 hours)
- Salt
- 1 small cup vinegar
- 1/2 tbsp Angelica powder

Method

Cover broad beans with double the amount of water in a big pot. Cook on a medium heat for around three hours, checking and giving them a stir every 15 minutes. Add more water as needed.

Cooking time will depend on the texture of the broad beans – for some reason some broad beans cook faster than others.

Once broad beans are soft enough to eat, drain them. Add vinegar and salt to serve.

Plate up and serve with the same sauce as above (salt, Angelica powder and/or sumac and vinegar)

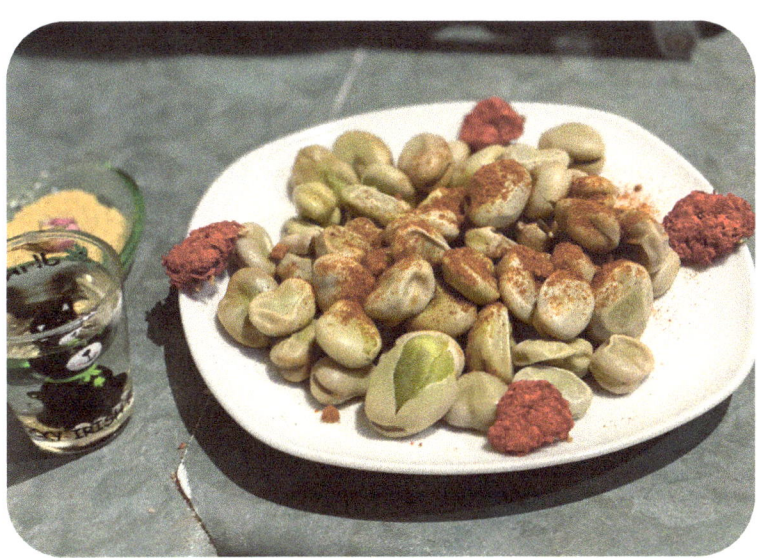

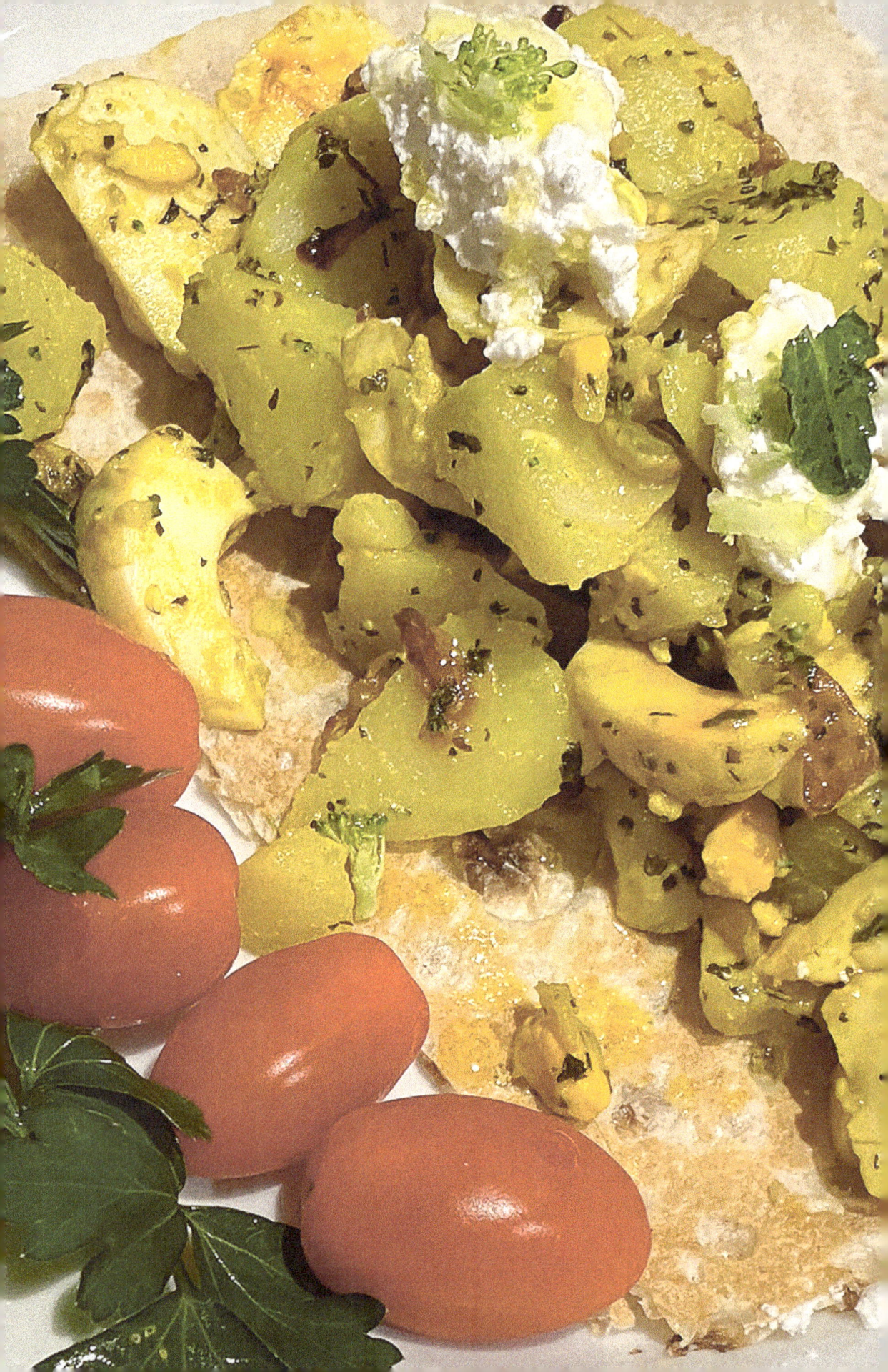

Yeralma Yumurta
(boiled potato and egg)

This particular street food might seem very simple yet it might be one of the oldest Iranian street foods due to its simple ingredients. Nearly 60 years ago, when Iranians had not been introduced to other cultural foods, it was the most popular sandwich. In fact, Iran's introduction to the sandwich started with this food: before, people would make a wrap with their leftovers and take it with them for their lunch or snack. Like the recipes above, it is more common in cold seasons.

Nowadays, with so many other foods – like falafel, other Turkish, Arabic even and Mexican street foods – joining the Iranian street food menu, this particular dish has fallen aside in most states. But it is still one of the favourites in many cities and the number one choice in the Oromiyeh province in the north west of Iran.

Passing through the streets of Oromiyeh (a city in North West), you will witness all sorts of vendors – either with old wooden wheelbarrows or even in shops – selling boiled potato and egg sandwiches. In fact, this food is one of the most famous tourist attractions in this area – like falafel, for Arabs.

There are two versions of this dish – with either boiled or baked potato, but the egg is always boiled. This dish comes with a big variety of sides, but the hero ingredients – potato and egg – are constantly acting in this scene. My recipe is a mix of both traditional and creative versions of this food.

There is very famous, historical park in Tabriz called Eel Goli, where there is a very interesting building in the middle of a big pool, which has been turned to a museum. Outside of this area, you will see all sorts of sellers selling this food. And that is the main market for this famous street food

Yet this building also has its own story. It used to be the king's summer residence. In the very old days when there was no systematic cooling equipment, people living in more modern areas like cities used to travel to cooler regional areas during this very part of summer. Usually, due to their work responsibilities, men would stay at home but the rest of the family would travel to these cooler places for a while. These cool places had to be close to the family's permanent residence so that the men could come and visit. As the working week started, they would return home to the city. So, this building Eel Goli used to be allocated for Qajar kings and their families, while the king's permanent residency was in the capital city.

When this dish is served on a wheelbarrow, the baked or boiled potato and egg are arranged in very neat patterns, like a pyramid, on top of each other on a big round tray. The heating system underneath the wheelbarrow not only keeps the food hot the whole day but creates a pleasant steam.

The potato and egg is always served on top of traditional bread, and will only come with western style bread if customers ask for it – and this makes the dish even more attractive. Eating these traditional foods in such places is not just about filling your tummy, but each step in the process of making these kinds of foods is like watching an interesting, exciting movie about the traditions of people you just met.

When you finish your wrap, you will be served hot, usually black, tea poured from tea pots and Samavar (old traditional tea serving equipment: small, thin, traditional glasses with designed saucers.

Serves 1

Cooking time (for baked potato): 30 minutes

Cooking time (with boiled potato): 20 minutes

- One potato
- One egg

Method

Cook the potato with skin on: either in the oven with salt, butter or oil (in this case boil egg separate)

or boil in salted water and with the egg for 20 minutes. (Some believe cooking potato on small pebbles tastes even better. If using this method, cover the base of a big pot with small hard pebbles and bake the potato, brushed with salt and butter, on top of the pebbles, over a low heat.)

Peel the potato and egg (if you baked the potato, leave unpeeled as it's more delicious with the skin).

Place potato and egg in the middle of a big piece of buttered flatbread, big enough to wrap up.

Break potato and egg in pieces and if you like, top with coarsely chopped fresh coriander, parsley and chives, thin slice of tomato, cucumber pickles and feta, cumin and Angelica powder. Flatten the mixture down, wrap it up and enjoy!

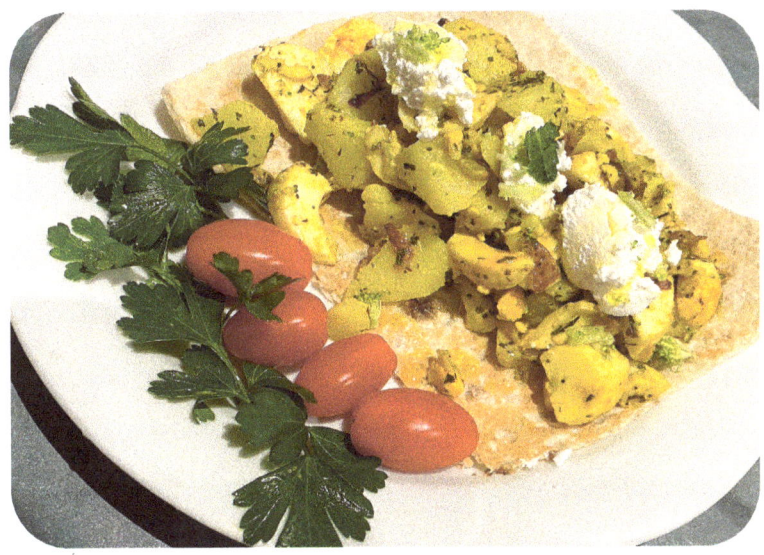

Local food

I might sound like I'm exaggerating if I say there's hardly a country in the world with as big a variety of local food as Iran – but this is true. If you consider the variety of climates in Iran and the fact that every local adjusts their food based on their climate, you may believe what I just said.

This big variety also makes it pretty hard to choose the best among the local foods: each one of them expresses the identity of their own state.

Being a happy tourist is not just limited to visiting a country's famous places; you can't be satisfied with your trip unless try the local foods. This food tells you something beyond its taste

Here, I introduce you to the most famous local Iranian foods: those which are not only famous in their own states but familiar to people in in other parts of the country, too.

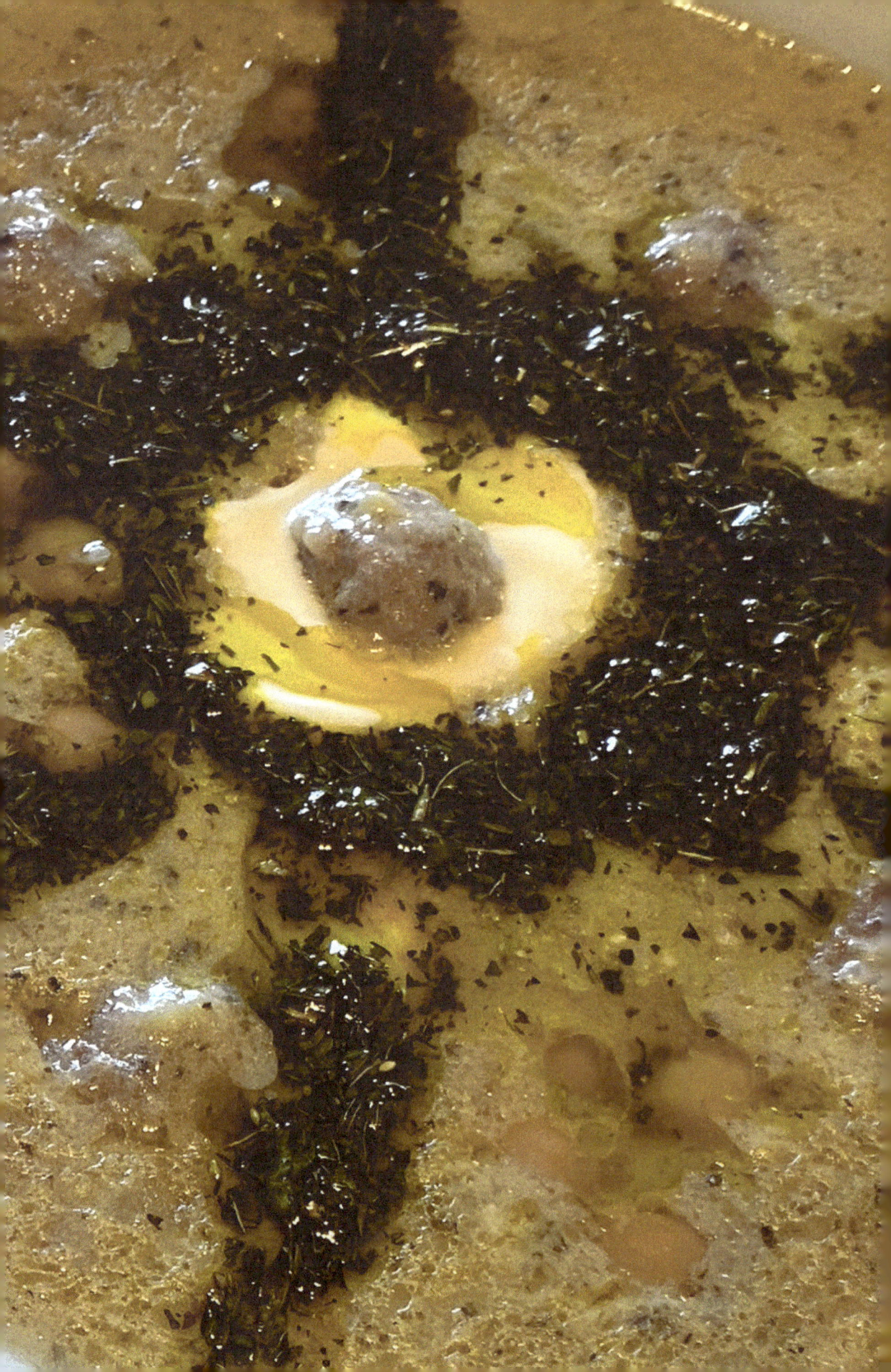

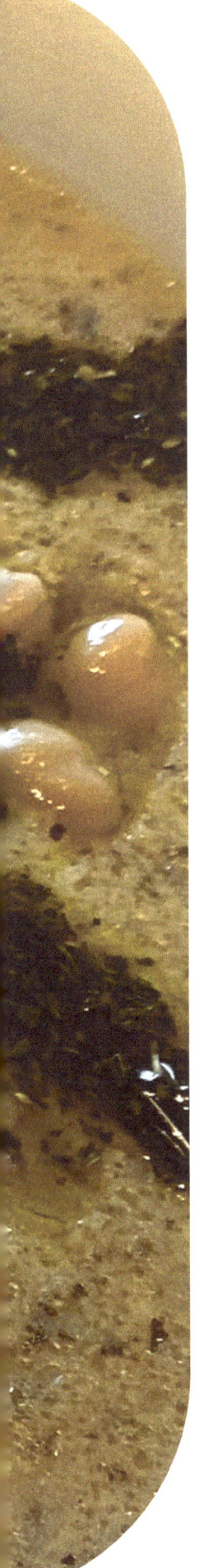

Ash-e Doogh
(thin yogurt soup)

Any soupy food in Persian is called 'ash' and there is a huge variety of ash in Persian food. Some are common to all states and some are originally from one particular state and are now eaten throughout the country.

Searching through Persian proverbs and slang, there is a lot of slang featuring the word 'ash', which proves how deeply this food is tied to Persian culture.

Some types of ash have religious backgrounds – as they were cooked for religious ceremonies but it's fascinating taste led them to be used during the rest of the year too. Among these, some, like ash-e doogh (thin yogurt soup) have become very popular in the past few decades.

Ash-e doogh is the signature dish for people who live in the north west of Iran. This is a very cold, mountainous area with cool, pleasant summers which makes this food desirable year-round, even in summertime. Traditionally, people working on farms in the cold weather needed something to fill them up and to warm up their body up at the same time. What made this soup even more popular was its use of local wild, aromatic herbs growing in the mountains. This recipe uses more well-known herbs in place of these special wild herbs.

If you travel by car to this area, you will see people selling this soup by the roadside. Imagine driving along a remote road and seeing someone in middle of that remote, regional area offering you soup (usually) cooked on wood!

Nowadays, you can find this soup in every house in Iran in the cold season. If served warm enough in cold winter's day, it will knock the socks right off your chilly little feet. It's also full of calcium.

There is also a Turkish version for this soup, and like every other common food shared between countries, both countries claim to be the origin of this soup.

If you're having it for first time, I suggest having just a small bowl until you get familiar with the sour, but pleasant taste of cooked yogurt.

Serves 8

Prep time: 15 minutes

Cooking time: 45 minutes

- 250 grams minced beef
- 1/2 onion, grated and drained
- 1/2 teaspoon salt plus more to taste
- 1/2 teaspoon black pepper
- 1/2 cup sticky or short grain rice (not long grain basmati)
- 1 egg
- 5 cups yogurt (mixed with 7.5 cups of water and 1/2 tsp salt until you get to a thin yogurt – this is called doogh – a middle eastern drink usually served with their food)
- 1 large bunch coriander, well washed and chopped
- 1 large bunch parsley, well washed and chopped
- 1 large bunch spring onions, well washed and chopped
- 1 medium tin chickpeas or 1/2 cup cooked chickpeas

- 1 tbsp dried mint
- 2 tbsp vegetable oil
- 2 heads of garlic, peeled and coarsely chopped
- 1 tsp dried thyme

Method

Combine minced beef, grated and drained onion, salt and pepper. Roll into small meatballs and set aside.

Break egg into the uncooked rice in a small bowl. Whisk well and set aside

Pour dough (thin yogurt) into a big pot over a low heat. Keep an eye on the pot, stirring with a wooden spoon, leaving wooden spoon in the pot to stop the pot from overflowing.

Add rice and egg mixture to the pot, and gradually increase the heat.

Add the meatballs to the soup.

Stir as you bring to the boil (about 20 minutes). After 2 minutes of boiling, reduce to medium heat and stir every few minutes.

Without removing the wooden spoon, add the herbs and spring onions. Continue to stir occasionally.

While stirring, add the chickpeas.

Simmer on a low heat and give a gentle stir occasionally.

Crush the dried mint in your hand and quickly fry in vegetable oil (10 seconds on the heat is enough to maintain the green colour – mint burns fast and colour goes dark easily).

Two minutes before serving, add the garlic.

Serve into bowls and garnish with fried mint and a pinch of dried thyme.

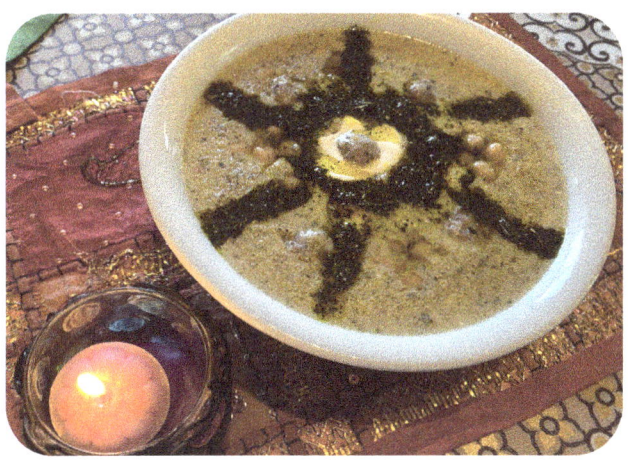

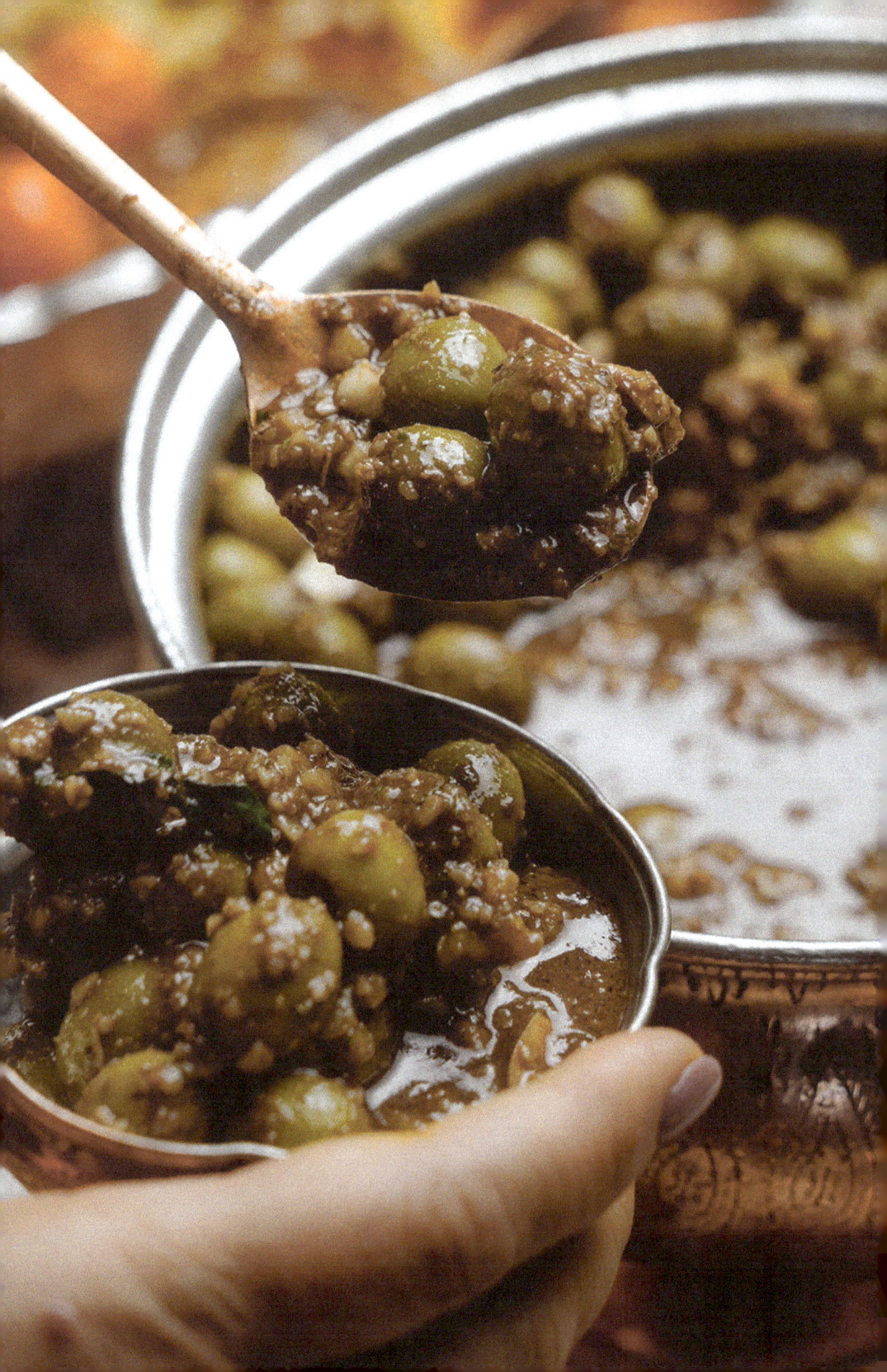

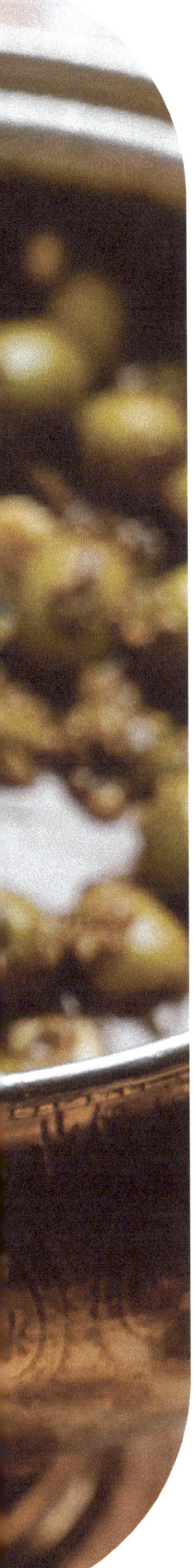

Zeytoon parvardeh
processed olive from north of Iran

There are few state in Iran which are blessed with very much greens.

And northern part of Iran is one of them in fact it's the greenest part of Iran, it's famous because of jungles, it's pleasant climate which is not very cold in most seasons and it's food which is totally different with other states when it comes to enjoying vacation, Northern area always is the first option not only because of its green location and pleasant weather but because it's close to Caspian Sea which share border with Soviet Union of Russia and people can enjoy swimming in sea which is not possible in other states.

Every summer time people who live in Northern area have lots of visitors and tourists and because of this reason tourism industry have prospered in this area more than any other place in Iran.

They not only have very well introduced their food and culture to residents from other states but also they have opportunity to show and sell their wide range of handcrafts such as Mat weaving which is so versatile in colour and texture.

It's interesting to know people in northern area love eating rice. Rice is the dominated food on their daily food intake and in most places, they even have cooked rice in morning instead of bread.

Nearly 30 years ago not in every suburb you were able to find a good bakery baking good quality bread. Visitors and tourists to this area used to advise each other if you're travelling there for any period of time, to take your bread with you. Because even if you find a bakery baking bread, their quality is not as good as other states. It's like people in these areas had an opinion that bread is not a necessity in daily food.

But nowadays as I said, thanks to the tourism industry growing hugely in these areas, if you travel there you will be able to find good quality bread.

Most foods in this area are plant-based and almost every one is growing their own vegetables and have their chocks in their backyard.

That makes cooking a very cost effective process for them as well as healthy and more delicious since every ingredient are usually freshly picked and it's organic for sure.

I remember especially when I was kid, before I fell in trap of work and daily life responsibilities, I used to travel to the Northern area with my parents.

Almost everybody else does the same summer when weather is more pleasant there .

North of Iran is a temple of joy and happiness for everyone all around other states.

Huge number of songs and movies have been made about this area and for all Iranian who have migrated to other countries if you ask what they have missed a lot about their homeland they all agree and will tell you it's travelling with their family to north of Iran.

Their food is so tasty and unforgettable in flavour.

The ingredients are usually very simple you can't believe at the end these simple ingredients turn to an art craft, like a famous artist using just a pen and piece of paper delivering it to a master piece.

As I said there are lots of jungle and green areas in north of Iran so in old days when people used to be very poor especially during war time they used to go for walking in jungle and pick whatever was eatable and turn it to a dish to feed the family.

Zeytoon Parvardeh (proceed olive) is one of those improvised dishes based on situation and ability. Since all the ingredients to bring a dish to plate was available in jungles.

I can say for sure Zeytoon Parvardeh is one of the most famous side dishes from north part of Iran but for me specially it has more meaning.

It reminds me of smile and cuddles I used to receive from of my auntie.

She was from northern states of Iran and back then not many people knew this dish.

It was not like today that if you step in to any good restaurant this is one of most wanted appetiser in their menu and everyone all around the country know it and have tasted it but those days the only place we could get and enjoy tastes for northern dish was in my auntie home.

For me that I was raised with no mother she and her food was scent of love.

There is not even one house or restaurant in northern states that they don't serve Zeytoon Parvaneh (processed olive) these days.

The unique taste not only comes from ingredients but also comes from the process that these ingredients are well combined together.

It's good to know when preparation is done and the dish is ready the best taste and flavour comes out of it if you leave it in fridge for few days before using it .

I must say that marriage between hospitality and generosity that Iranian people are famous for around the world and specially it's true for people who live in Northern states is another point that makes all Persian dishes more tasty.

But special thing for this dish has for me comes from feelings that my auntie used to give me by preparing this dish for me.

Everyone needs to feel special in life sometimes and for me this feeling only happened when my auntie used to say if you be a good girl I make you some Zeytoon Parvaneh.

There is not even a single day that I forget my home land with all those sad or happy memories but when I'm making this dip it really makes me time travel, makes me smile while I'm preparing it because it not only tastes like home but it also tastes like love.

Processed olive or Zeytoon Parvardeh

A taste from Persia

Made with olive and pomegranate molasses

Serves: 8

Preap time: 20 minutes

- 2 jar of medium pitted green olives coarsely chopped
- 1/2 cup extra virgin olive oil
- 1 1/2 cup well ground walnut and 2 coarsely chopped and few walnut for garnish
- 1/4 cup pomegranate molasses with 1/4 cup of pomegranate seeds for garnish
- 1/4 cup fresh chopped mint
- 2 gloves of chopped garlic (in original recipe there is no garlic but by experiencing I found out garlic can add the taste and flavour you can skip if you don't like the taste of garlic in this appetiser)
- 1 table spoon of balsamic vinegar
- 1/2 teaspoon ground dry or fresh thyme

Again in the very original recipe what is really prepared by northern residents is wild local herbs which they pick by hand from the jungles. But even in other states of Iran you can't find the original herbs as they only grew wild in northern jungles so we replaced them with mint and thyme.

Those magical herbs are very much aromatic and I only found these two herbs aroma close to the actual herbs used in the original recipe. If you used can olive which is easier and much more accessible you don't need salt otherwise use salt and pepper for your taste.

Method

Combine chopped garlic, dry thyme powder, chopped mint and thyme (locals used regional herbs) chopped walnut in a mixing bowl.

Gradually stir and add in the pomegranate molasses, then stir in olive oil and balsamic vinegar (lemon juice), mix well to form a thick paste.

Then add coarsely chopped olive and pomegranate molasses and pomegranate seeds stir gently to incorporate.

Transfer to a jar with tight fitting lid, seal and could be refrigerated. It won't go off and could be saved in fridge For more than 10 days.

Best way to use is as it could be eaten with either flat bread or crackers as dip.

Or as side for any dish , add to give more taste to any kind of salad or served as an appetiser.

When left in fridge pls bring to room temperature before using.

If you can't wait long For best result I suggest to make at least 2 hours hours before using it.

Noosh E Jan (Bonna petit in Persian)

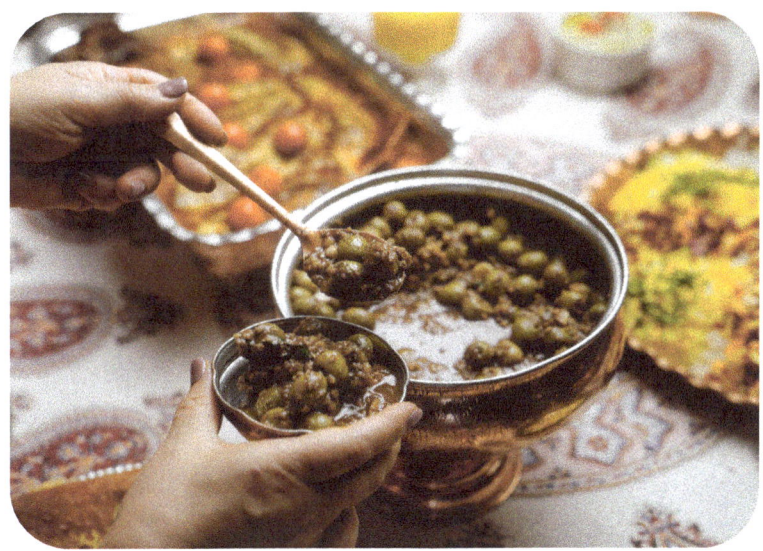

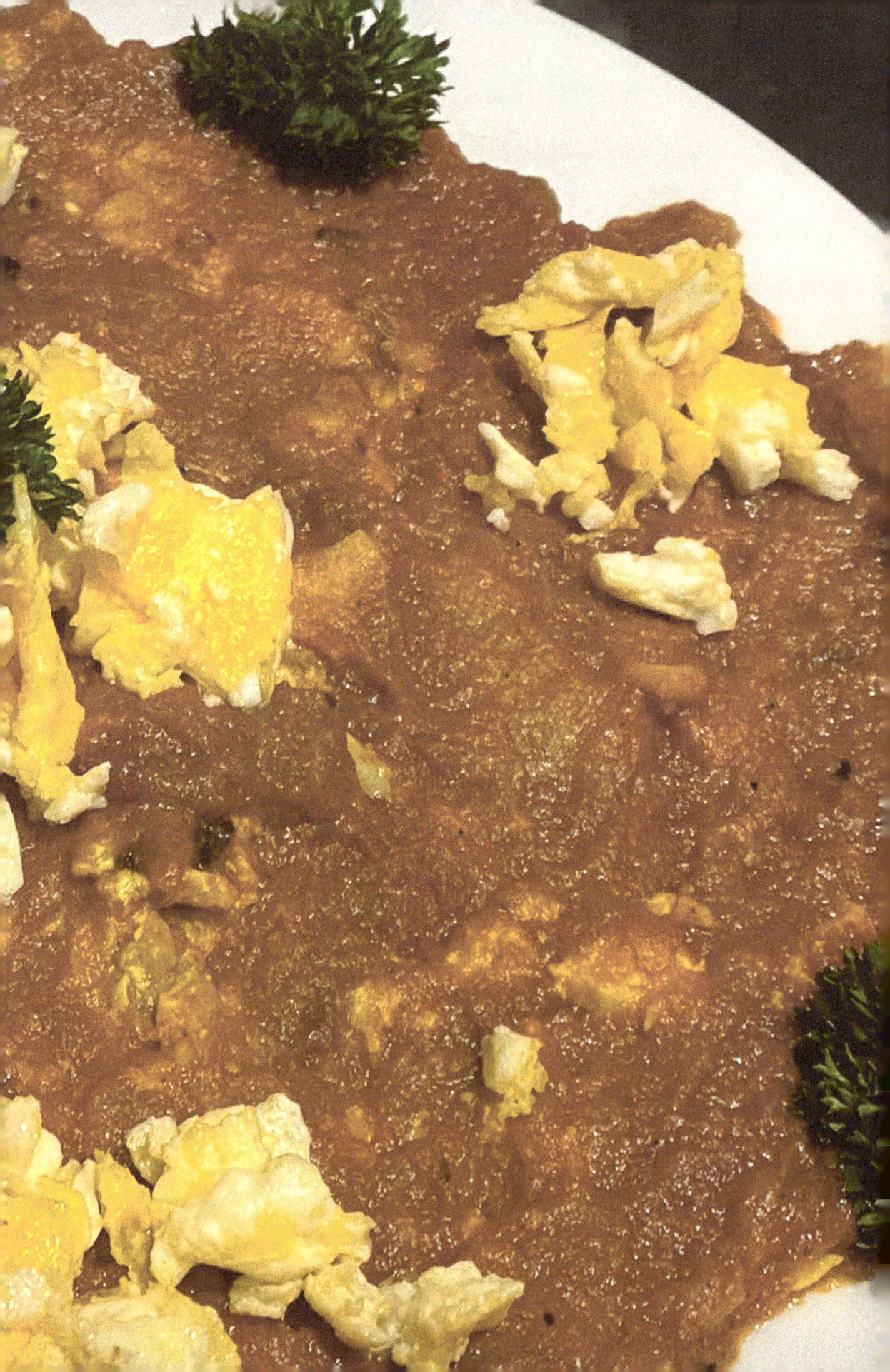

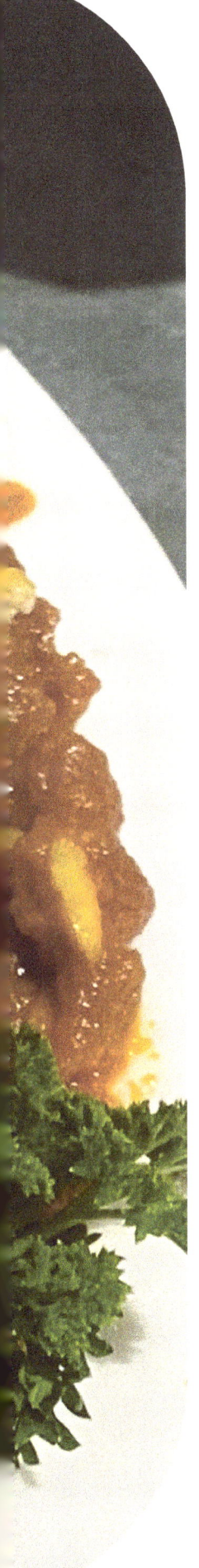

Mirza Ghasemi
(smoked eggplant with garlic and egg)

Very well known all over the country, Mirza Ghasemi is a dip, served with flatbread, or with plain rice as lunch or dinner.

Mirza Ghasemi is originally from northern Iran, a very green area with high chances of rain during year. This not only makes this area very beautiful but the most popular tourist destination among Iranians. When people travel to northern Iran more than anywhere else in country, obviously they know about its food more than any other states in Iran. For this reason, this area's local foods are the most familiar local foods to other states. They are also amazingly delicious, mostly plant-based with as little as spice – especially hot spice – as possible.

Almost all food in northern Iran features garlic as the hero ingredient since it's believed that living in a humid state will impact on your muscles, and eating garlic daily will kill this negative side effect.

Another interesting thing about northern Iran is that almost everybody grows their own vegetables in their backyard.

So homegrown vegetables are probably the first choice of food if you just drop into local people's houses unexpectedly. Another thing about Iranians is – no matter if they expected you or not – if you knock on their door for any reason, they will strongly insist you stay for food. In fact, not insisting unexpected guests stay for lunch or dinner is a sign of humiliation for that guest.

Mirza Ghasemi is the only Persian food named after a man. Mirza Mohamad Ghasem was governor of Gillan province (not everybody had chance to study those days, so people who were able to read and write used to be called Mirza. Mirza was not only a title but also could be job too. Mirza people used to illiterate charge people to do their paperwork).

Anyway, surprisingly, our Mirza was very much a fan of cooking too. Surprisingly because first, he was a man and second, he was governor. It was not common for a man in his position to go into the kitchen and start cooking. He loved to try cooking new dishes and invented this dish, which is named after him.

Like many other regional foods, it's only in past few decades that people have started knowing about other states food rather than just practicing their normal routine menu.

These days, if you drop into any Persian restaurant this is the first dish offered but it definitely wasn't like that forty years ago.

This healthy, nutritious and yet very tasty Persian dish – ideal as an entree or a very tasty vegetarian dish – with soft smoked or roasted eggplant in tomato and garlic sauce takes you to heaven.

There are big variety of recipes from northern Iran featuring eggplant as the hero ingredient. People from this part of the country have a proverb which says that the taste of eggplant can compare with taste of chicken: they call it the black chicken that can't walk. This poetic slang, when said in a strong local accent, is even more interesting.

Serves 4

Prep time: 30 minutes

Cooking time: 45 minutes

- 3 large eggplants
- 1 cup vegetable oil, for frying
- Cloves of 1 whole garlic, peeled and thinly sliced

- 1/2 tsp turmeric
- 3 large tomatoes or 1 tin tomato purée
- 2 tbsp tomato paste
- 1 tbsp salt
- 2 eggs
- Walnut, for garnishing

Method

Blister whole eggplants over an open flame. Pierce each eggplant in a few places to allow the extra water to exit by the time the eggplants start smoking. (You can roast eggplants in the oven too but smoked flavour of eggplant really make big difference on taste).

The eggplants are ready when their skins are blackened and flesh is soft through to the centre. We are looking for super soft flesh on the eggplants.

Set aside to cool – ideally in a bowl with glad wrap on top. This will make it easier to remove the skin from the eggplants when they have cooled down.

When the eggplants have cooled down, take off the glad wrap and gently take off the blackened skin with your fingers, Do not use running water at this stage – the skin might come off easily under running water but the smoked flavour, which is the secret to the interesting flavour for this dish, will be gone. Later, chop the eggplant flesh finely.

Heat vegetable oil in a large frying pan on a medium heat. Add garlic and stir. Before they are brown, add the fresh or tinned tomatoes and the chopped eggplant. Give a good stir.

Add turmeric, tomato paste and salt, stir well for 7 to 8 minutes until all extra water is evaporated. Reduce the heat, and gently move the mixture into one side of the pan, leaving the other side empty.

Break the eggs into the empty side of the pan and mix like a scrambled egg until it starts to hold together.

Mix the egg into the rest of the mixture and continue to cook on a low heat for few minutes.

Dish up, and garnish with chopped walnuts and fresh herbs. For garnish some fry another egg separately, serve it on top of the Mirza Ghasemi and eat it with flatbread as dip or plain rice as main,

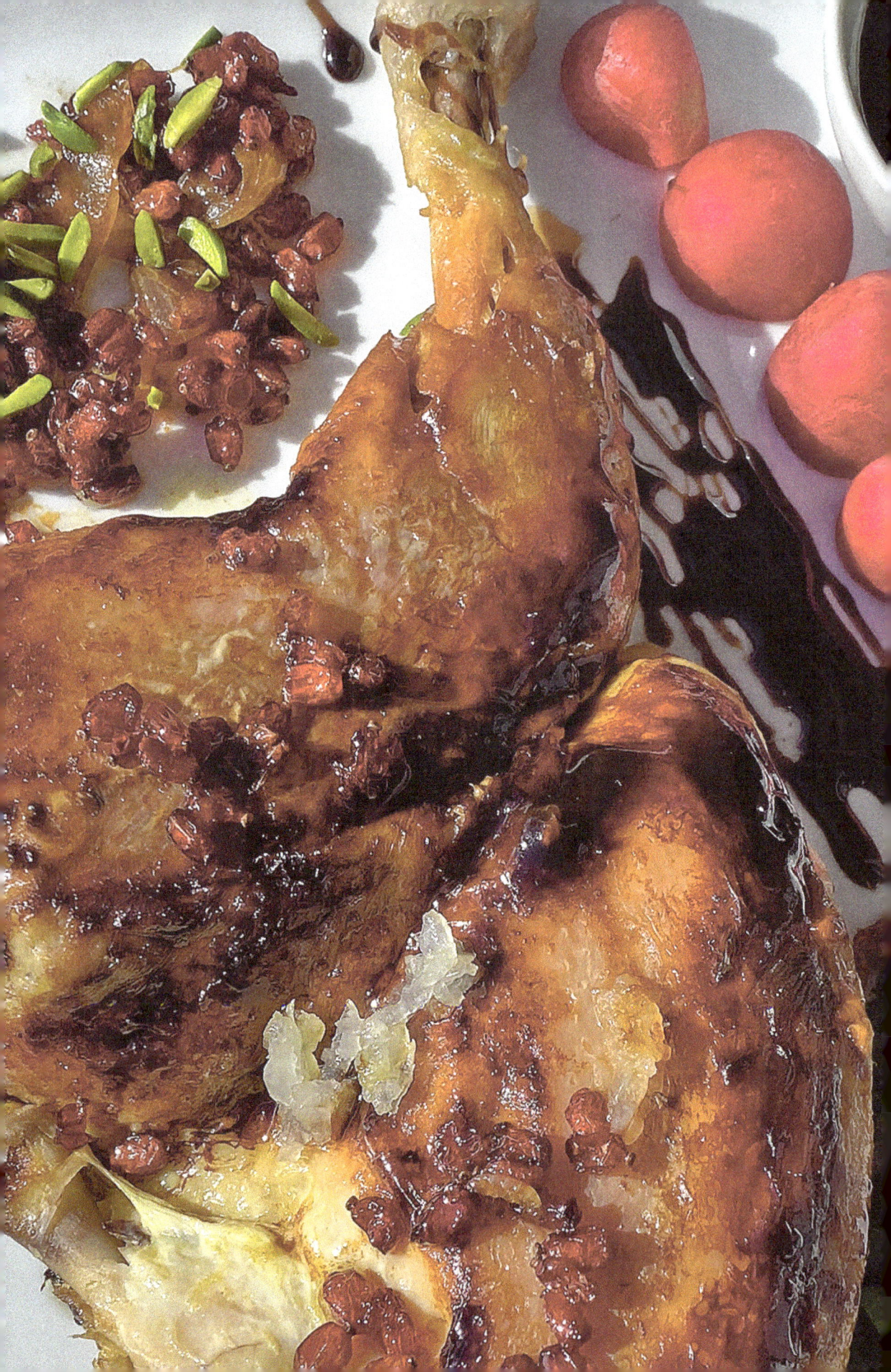

- 1/2 tsp turmeric
- 3 large tomatoes or 1 tin tomato purée
- 2 tbsp tomato paste
- 1 tbsp salt
- 2 eggs
- Walnut, for garnishing

Method

Blister whole eggplants over an open flame. Pierce each eggplant in a few places to allow the extra water to exit by the time the eggplants start smoking. (You can roast eggplants in the oven too but smoked flavour of eggplant really make big difference on taste).

The eggplants are ready when their skins are blackened and flesh is soft through to the centre. We are looking for super soft flesh on the eggplants.

Set aside to cool – ideally in a bowl with glad wrap on top. This will make it easier to remove the skin from the eggplants when they have cooled down.

When the eggplants have cooled down, take off the glad wrap and gently take off the blackened skin with your fingers, Do not use running water at this stage – the skin might come off easily under running water but the smoked flavour, which is the secret to the interesting flavour for this dish, will be gone. Later, chop the eggplant flesh finely.

Heat vegetable oil in a large frying pan on a medium heat. Add garlic and stir. Before they are brown, add the fresh or tinned tomatoes and the chopped eggplant. Give a good stir.

Add turmeric, tomato paste and salt, stir well for 7 to 8 minutes until all extra water is evaporated. Reduce the heat, and gently move the mixture into one side of the pan, leaving the other side empty.

Break the eggs into the empty side of the pan and mix like a scrambled egg until it starts to hold together.

Mix the egg into the rest of the mixture and continue to cook on a low heat for few minutes.

Dish up, and garnish with chopped walnuts and fresh herbs. For garnish some fry another egg separately, serve it on top of the Mirza Ghasemi and eat it with flatbread as dip or plain rice as main,

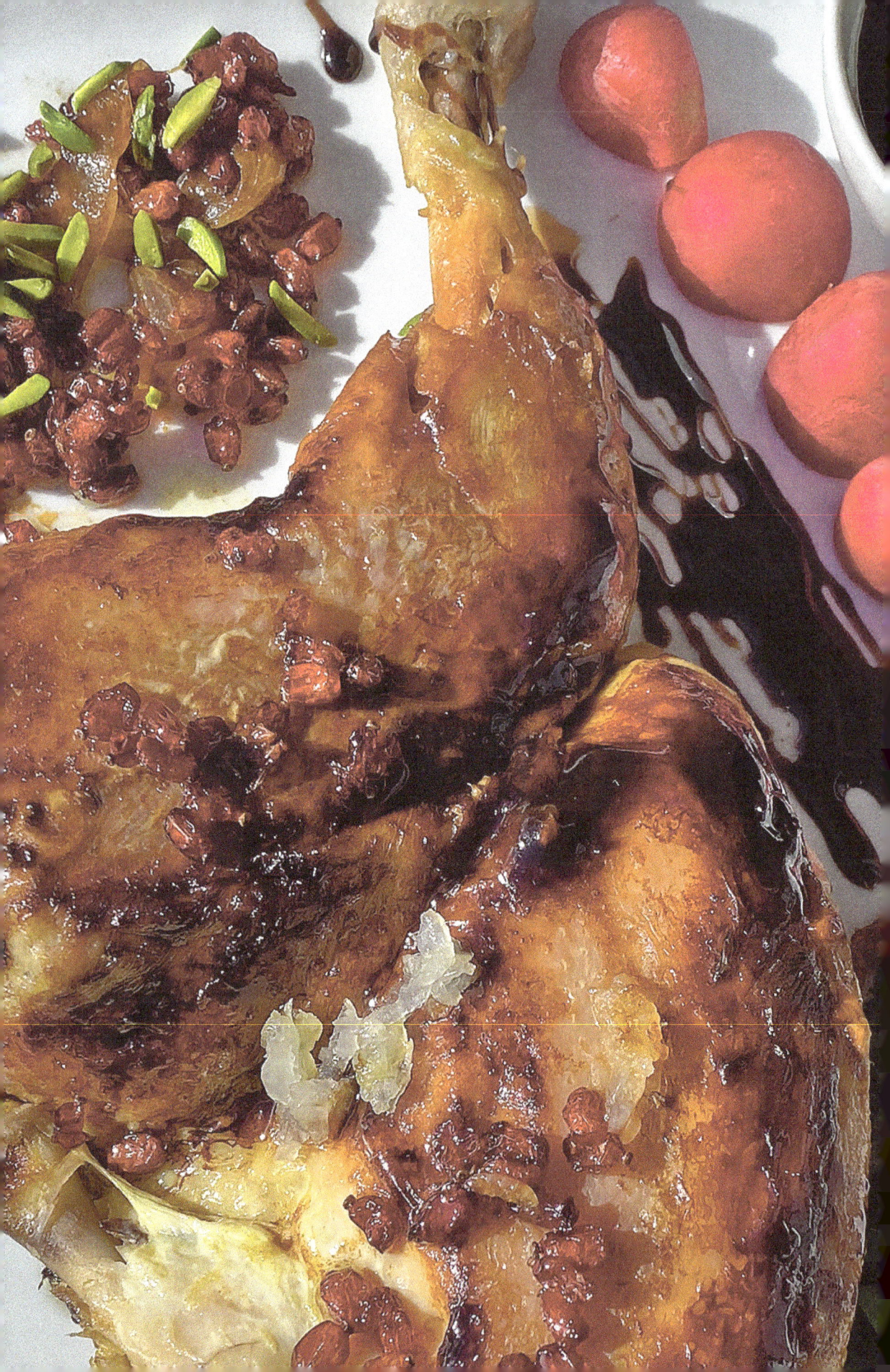

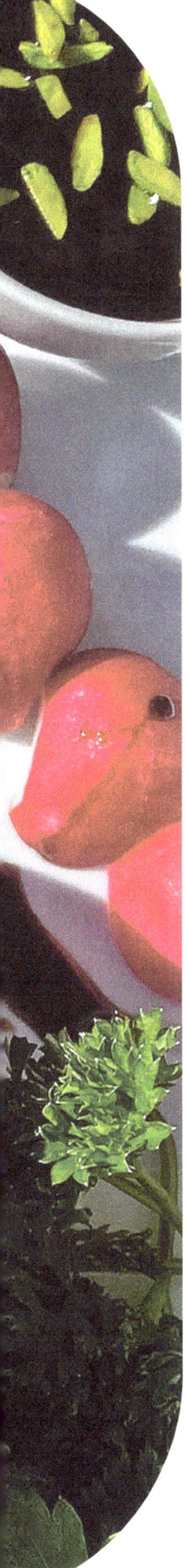

Akbar Joheh
(Akbar chicken)

There is a road between a province in northern Iran and the religious city of Mashhad, which pilgrims to Mashad must pass to get to their destination. There are lots of teahouses and roadside restaurants in this place.

In 1945, one of these small teahouses belonged to a man named Akbar Kalbadi Nejad, who ran the teahouse with his wife. Compared to other teahouse, their tea house was very small, with very little income. So, Akbar also used to cook pomegranate paste made from the garden behind their teahouse to help raise their income.

Akbar was also a great cook. Together with his wife, he invented a new method of cooking chicken with a different marinade, that no one had ever tasted before. He deep fried his marinated chickens in big pot full of melted butter and served the chickens with a special sauce made from their own homemade pomegranate paste and saffron rice. Soon, customers were lined up in front of their teahouse to try this new recipe.

That road was always full of cars and buses passing by and since Akbar's prices were the most reasonable among all the other teahouses along the road, soon he and his new food were famous. More and more, people started asking for this new chicken recipe. And because it was distinguished from other restaurants and teahouses' food, they called it Akbar Jojeh (Akbar chicken).

Soon, Akbar's teahouse was not big enough to serve all of these customers. The demand for Akbar Jojeh was so high that he opened another bigger restaurant, and another and another, all serving only Akbar Jojeh with its special pomegranate side sauce and saffron rice.

Nowadays, this recipe is served by restaurants and teahouses all over Iran, but especially in northern Iran where there are lots of roadside restaurants and teahouses. They all serve Akbar Jojeh as one of the main dishes on their menus. Some have tried different marinades or different side sauces but the original recipe is still the best, in the highest demand from customers. This one recipe made Akbar a very wealthy man and now, people repeat his name every day in restaurants around the country. Now his grandchildren are running his restaurants but everyone else also knows about this food.

Serves 2

Prep time: 12 hours for marinade

Cooking time: 3 hours 20 minutes

- One chicken (between 700–800 grams or even less is better)
- 1/4 cup brewed saffron
- 150 grams butter
- 1 large onion
- 4 cloves garlic
- 1/2 cup lemon juice
- 1/2 cup pomegranate paste or molasses
- 2 tbsp extra lemon juice for sauce
- 2 tbsp crushed walnuts
- 1 tbsp olive oil
- Salt and pepper as needed
- Vegetable oil as needed, for deep frying

Method

Remove as much skin as you can from the chicken and wash and dry.

Cut the chicken in half lengthways.

Peel onion and garlic. Coarsely chop them both and add salt and pepper.

Add brewed saffron and lemon juice to the onion and garlic and rub over all sides of the halved chicken.

Mix well, and leave in fridge for at least for 12 hours or if you can, overnight.

Heat vegetable in a big, deep pot (as much as needed to cover chicken with oil).

When oil is hot enough, place each half of the chicken in the pot. When the colour of the chicken starts to change, put the lid on the pot and lower the heat to a minimum.

Cook the chicken for around 45 minutes.

When the chicken is cooked, remove from the oil and stir fry it in butter for five more minutes.

To make the sauce, or molasses: either serve the chicken with plain pomegranate paste or mix every 4 tablespoons of pomegranate paste with two tablespoons of lemon juice and 1 tablespoon of olive oil, one clove of grated garlic and two table tablespoons of crushed walnuts.

Serve with saffron rice.

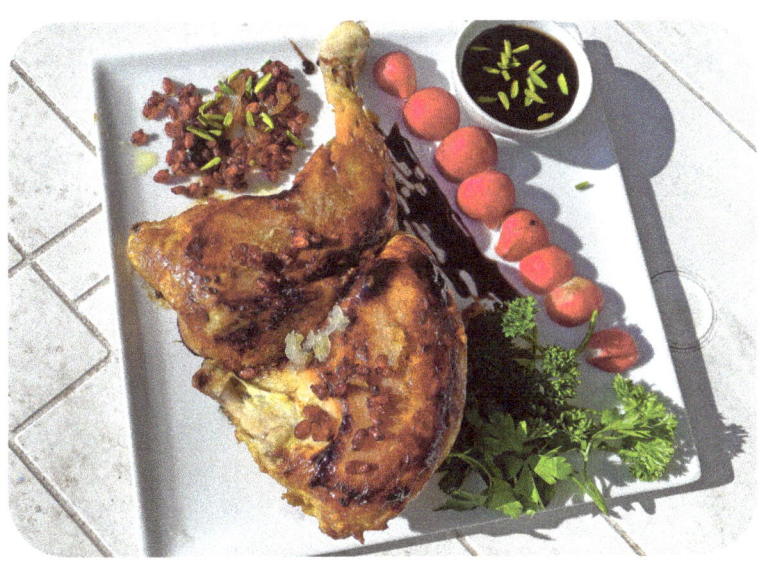

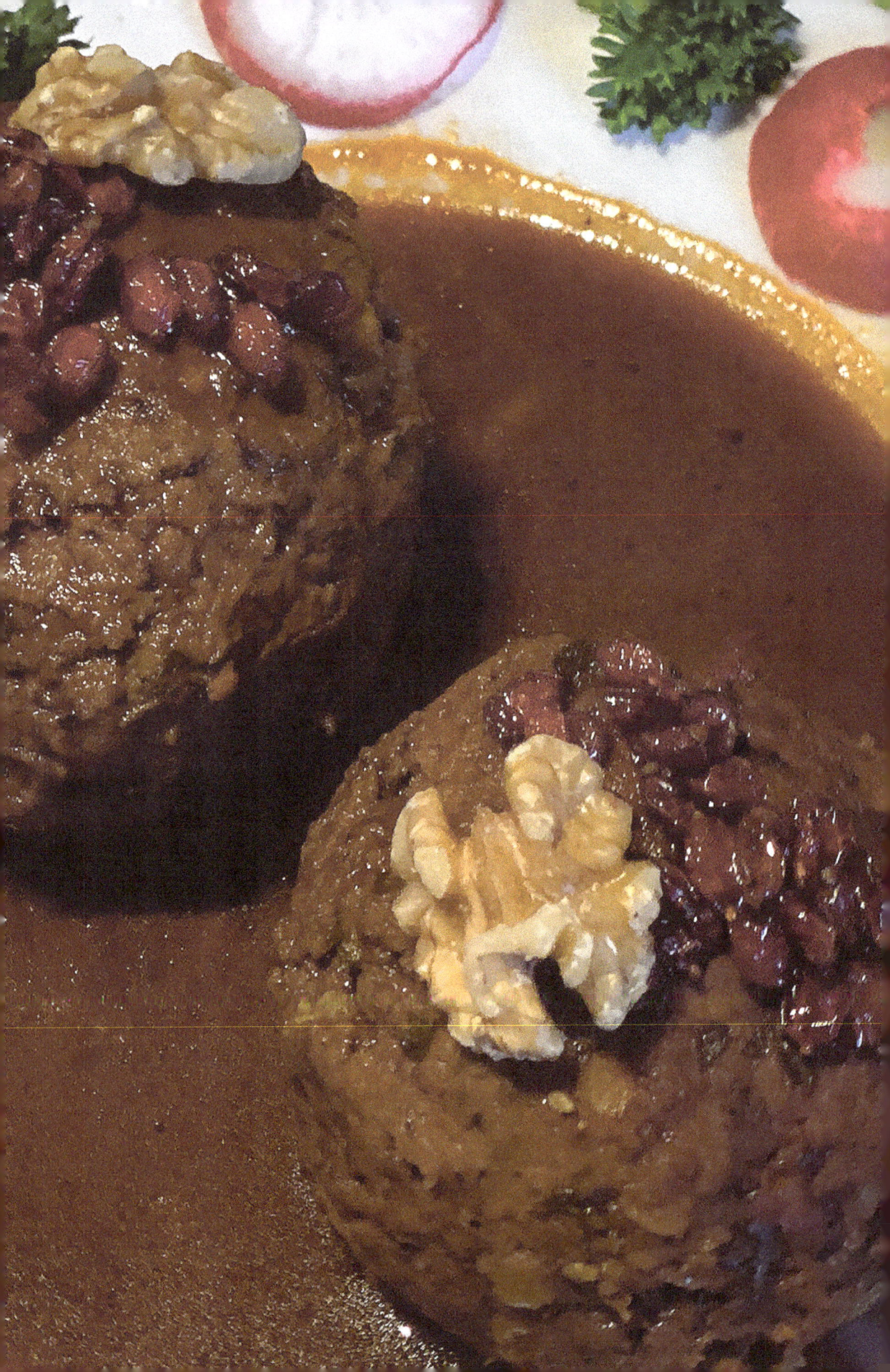

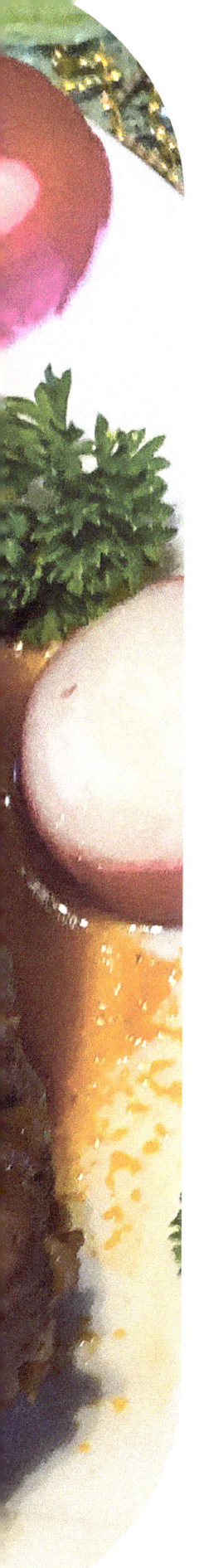

Kofteh tabrizi
(juicy meatballs with herbs and lentil)

Kofteh (meatballs) is a common dish between Iranian, Greek and Turkish people – but Persian kofteh is totally different from the others.

Like so many dishes from Iran, there is a big variety of kofteh in Persian food, but the most famous one is from city of Tabriz. We already talked about one of most famous street foods – boiled potato and egg – which is originally from Tabriz and other neighbouring cities like Oromiyeh. Kofteh Tabrizi is even more famous than this street food. When a food is named after a city it should be cooked well, with consideration for the reputation of that city. Unlike Greek and Turkish kofteh, the Persian version of kofteh is big and juicy.

In some versions of kofteh Tabrizi, the kofteh is as big as a soccer ball – this is the hardest version to cook in a way that it won't lose its shape. In some other versions, which are easier to prepare, the kofteh are more like the size of mandarins. If the kofteh are as big as a soccer ball, one is enough for the whole family and if smaller, one for each member of the family is enough. In my cooking classes, I usually I teach the smaller version, since the smaller the size the less chance the kofteh will fall apart. Even women who have been cooking Persian food for long time are still stressed to cook kofteh Tabrizi since there is a big chance they will fall apart while they are cooking. So, you really need some special techniques and a few secret hacks to save your kofteh from falling apart. But even if they do – don't worry, you're still going to have a very tasty thick soup, which will taste like kofteh (even if it doesn't look like kofteh!)

So why is this dish named after Tabriz? Tabriz is a very famous historical city in the north west of Iran. Many political protests through history have started from Tabriz, so it is a very important city in this sense as well. It's also close to Russia and its culture and traditions are influenced by this special geographical position.

Tabriz is also very cold through most of the year. This climate leads people in this part of Iran to eat more soupy kinds of food. While not a soup, the thick sauce that comes with kofteh Tabrizi could almost fall into this category. People first eat the sauce in a bowl with broken pieces of flatbread soaked inside the sauce, and eating the kofteh, filled with nuts and dried fruit, second with pickles or fresh herbs.

Kofteh Tabrizi was also the favourite food of the last Iran king Mohammad Reza Shah, and his Mother, the queen Mother, used to cook it for him herself. I suppose she was the only queen in history that used to cook. But I guess that is just a sign of love between a mother and her child – even if you're a king and your mother is a queen who hardly lifts a finger throughout her days but enjoys cooking the king his favourite food with her own hands. Maybe this is the reason it is called king of foods in Tabriz.

Kofteh Tabrizi is considered more of a homemade than a restaurant food, but since it's very famous and almost a signature for this city, you will see a lot of restaurants in Tabriz serving it too. In Tehran, the capital city you can hardly find any restaurants serving Kofteh Tabrizi because, but in Tabriz the story is different.

The word Kofteh means smashed, as in the old days, they used to use a big stone mortar and pestle to ground meat. This was such a hard job – usually reserved for the younger people in the house – and on the days that women planned to cook with grounded meat they made sure they didn't have any other jobs to do that day.

There are some children's stories in Tabriz culture that repeat the name of kofteh tabrizi several times. Referring to very old traditional stories, these stories prove that having Kofteh in the history of Tabriz city goes back much further than we know.

These days, kofteh Tabrizi is registered as an intangible national heritage.

Serves 4

Cooking time: 3 hours
Prep time: 90 minutes

- 500 grams minced beef
- 1/2 cup split yellow lentils, cooked
- 1 medium onion, finely grated and drained
- 1 tbsp turmeric
- 1 tbsp dried tarragon
- 1/2 tbsp dried mint
- 1 tsp salt
- 1 tsp pepper
- Salt and black pepper
- 1/2 cup sticky or short grain rice, washed and soaked for at least two hours
- 1/2 cup fresh parsley, finely chopped
- 1/2 cup fresh coriander, finely chopped
- 1/2 cup fresh chives, finely chopped
- 1 tbsp flour
- 1 egg

For filling:

- Dried plums, one per meatball
- Half walnut per meatball
- 150 grams barberries

For sauce:

- 1/2 cup vegetable oil
- 2 large onions, chopped
- 1 tsp turmeric
- 1/2 cup tomato paste
- 3 tbsp fresh lemon juice
- 2 tbsp tamarind purée

Method

In a medium bowl, combine minced meat, cooked lentils, onion, turmeric, tarragon, mint, salt and pepper.

Drain soaked rice, mix well and add to above mixture.

Add the fresh chopped herbs. Mix all ingredients together, then add egg and flour.

Mix well with your hands or ideally, a food processor until you have a consistent texture. This part is very important to the kofteh keeping its shape while its cooking. If you're not feeling confident, use more meat than the rest of the ingredients – when you have more meat than other ingredients, this helps your kofteh to keep its shape when cooked.

Have a bowl of cold water next to you and use to wet your hands. Take some of the mixture (as big as a mandarin), flattening it roughly in your hand and setting the dried plum, walnut and a few barberries inside. Fold it well into the shape of a ball to ensure all of the filling is hidden inside your ball. Make sure there are no cracks in any sides of your kofteh. Repeat until you have used up all of the mixture (this recipe should makes approximately about 10 kofteh).

In a large pot, fry chopped onion until light golden brown. Add the rest of the turmeric, tomato sauce, lemon juice and tamarind purée. Mix well and fill a 1/3 of the pot with boiling water. Mix well and bring to the boiling.

Gently add your kofteh to the pot simmer on low–medium heat for three hours.

When the sauce reduced by half, the kofteh are done

As directed, first have the sauce with soaked broken pieces of bread and then the kofteh separately with any desired salad or pickles.

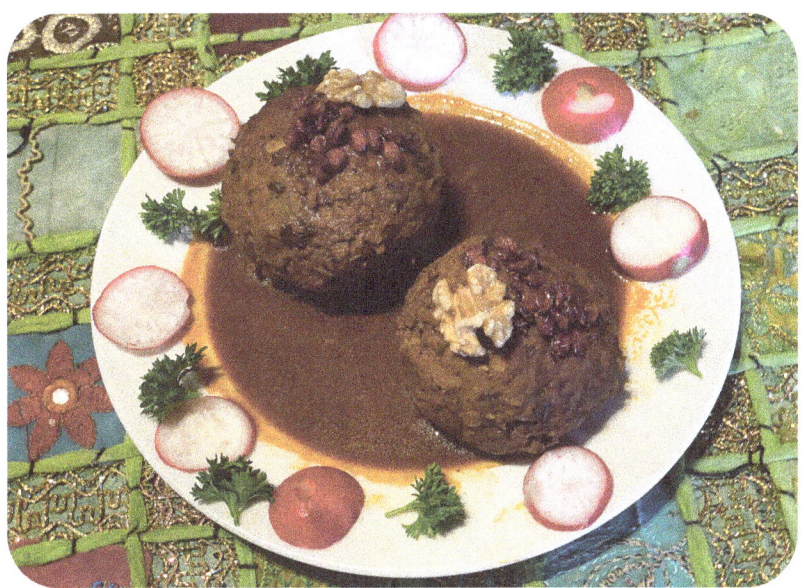

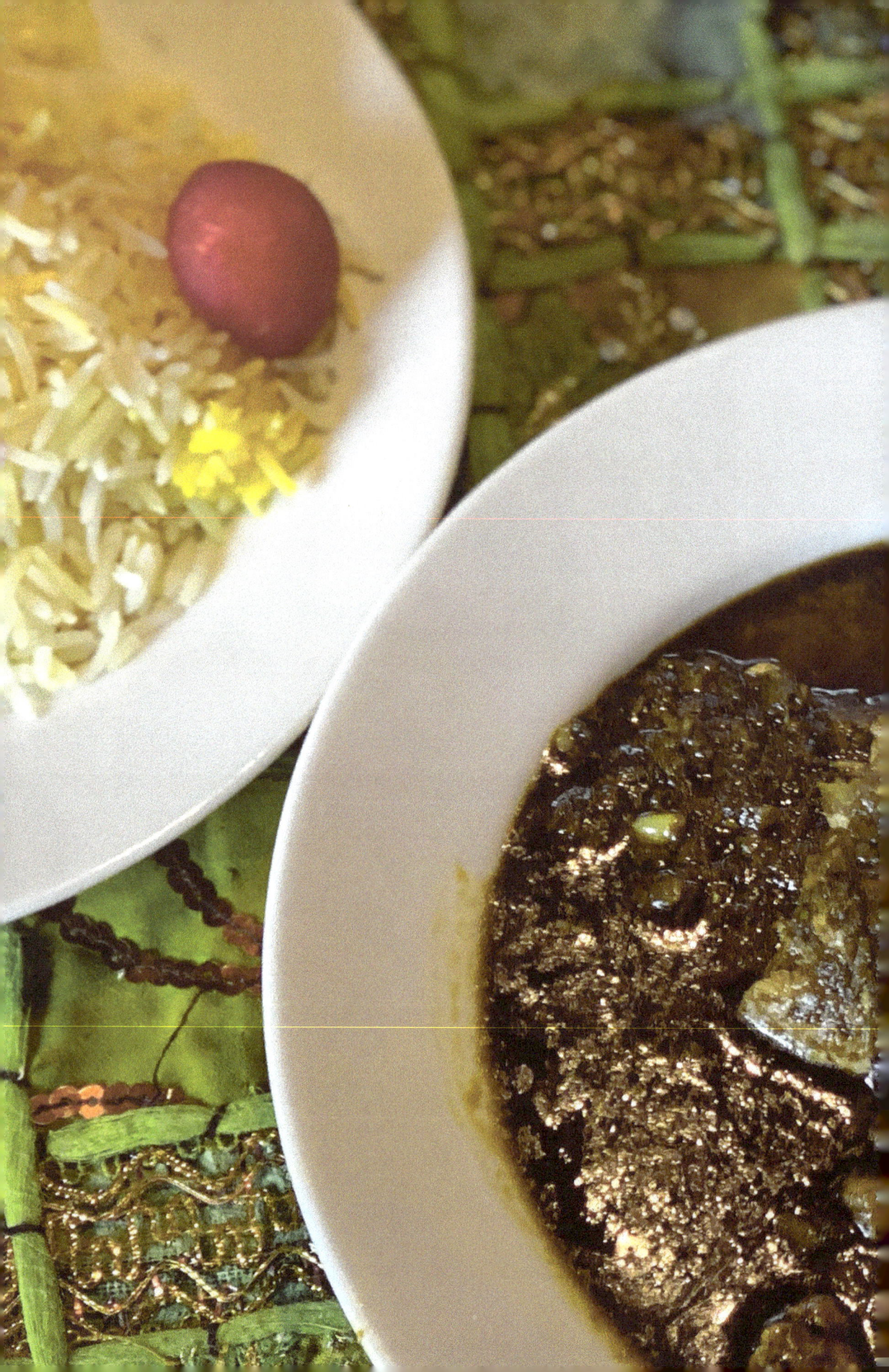

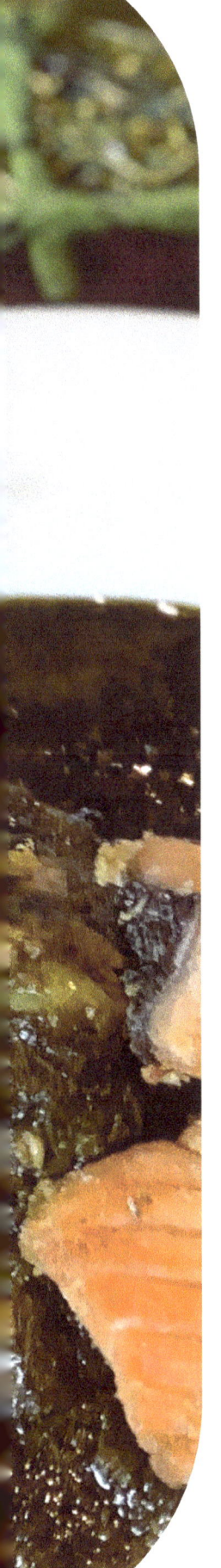

Ghalyeh Mahi
(fried fish stew in tamarind sauce)

Every city has its own signature dish that melts the hearts of its passengers, making them determined to travel there. In the southern states of Iran, although there are some very famous street foods, such as samosa, the most important local food is Ghalyeh Mahi: fried fish stew in tamarind sauce (ghalyeh means fried and mahi means fish).

The southern states are attached to the Persian Gulf (it's always Persian Gulf and no other name –Iranians are very prejudiced about this name) so there is a huge, advanced fishing industry in this area. Every evening, fisherman sell their daily catch in the fish market. For people from this part of Iran, although they are not fans of all kinds of seafoods, fish and shrimp are two key ingredients in their foods.

Surprisingly, this dish goes well with all sorts of fish and each southern city has its own favourite fish for this dish but the best kind of fish for this dish is usually used in the city of Booshehr. Some recipes use shrimp instead of fish, which cooks faster, but the best fish to use are those with more meat and less bones.

It is said that in the very old days, when fishing was not as technical and mechanised as it is today, it was hard for fishermen to catch fish. So, they decided to invent a recipe that allowed them to take advantage of whatever amount of fish they had caught that day.

There is one old very tradition among people living in the southern states: when you visit someone's home – no matter how many dishes they have already prepared for you – Ghalyeh Mahi will definitely be one of them. If you ever have the chance to travel to southern Iran, you're definitely going to be served by local people as their hospitality to travellers is very famous. Because there were also a lot of foreigners from western countries working in the oil refineries in these areas – local people were also the best English-speaking people in the country. Local people from this area of Iran are very generous and warm, and are famous for being happiest people among other states. Before the revolution in 1978, everywhere in the big southern cities you could see groups of boys carting portable stereos playing party music and dancing in the streets – this was a very normal scene, especially in the evenings after a day's work. Cities were alive 24/7.

But things have changed a lot since then. Dancing in the streets is now a big crime, since a religious, very restricted government is ruling in Iran. Still, these local people keep up with life and find other reasons to be happy – such as enjoying local food and family gatherings. Even in times of economic crisis, people in the south still have more family gatherings than any other states. At all of these gatherings, fish is a constant member at the table.

Even though people in this part of Iran suffered for eight years through the 1980s, living in very hard situations through the war between Iran and Iraq, they stood back on their feet again and to rebuild their homes which were all destroyed from bombing during the war. During the war, many left their homes to move to other safer, states. After the war, some came back but some have migrated forever. When they came back, they were faced with ghost towns. All of the famous palm trees in southern cities were beheaded.

The palm tree has very special place in the southern areas of Iran – here, they respect it and talk about it as if is a human being. Since if palm trees are cut from head they never grow again, southern people believe these trees are alive like humans. For this reason, in this area if someone cuts the head off a palm tree intentionally, this is considered a very big crime and has huge legal penalty. After the war, people started to build the city and plant new palm trees but they are not quite the same happy people again.

Still, southern people are famous for smiling in any rough and hard situation. They believe as they live in hot weather, their blood is warm too, and this helps them to keep cool through life's hard burdens. The long hot summers and short cold season, plus being close to Arabic countries has also affected people's daily life and habits – there are southern cities where people speak Arabic fluently as well as Farsi, and even dress like Arabs: these people are called Arabs from southern Iran. Of course, their eating habits are also highly influenced by Arabic recipes, and only in this part of country are people fans of highly spiced and hot food.

Serves 2

Cooking time: 2 hours

- 2 medium pieces of any fish filet
- 2 tbsp flour
- 1 tsp of turmeric
- Salt and black pepper
- 1 tsp of red chilli
- Vegetable oil, for frying
- 2 medium onion, finely diced
- 8 cloves garlic, finely minced
- 3 cups fresh coriander, chopped
- 1 cup of fresh fenugreek, chopped or 1/4 cup dried fenugreek
- 1 cup tamarind purée
- 1/3 cup lemon juice

Method

Combine flour with turmeric, salt and red chilli, generously coat the fish with this mixture. Set aside for 15 minutes.

Dust off any excess flour before frying the fish.

Heat 2 tablespoons of vegetable oil in a skillet on medium heat and lightly sauté the fish on all sides. Set aside.

In another large pan, fry the onion until the colour starts to change. Stir and add turmeric and chopped garlic and continue to stir fry for another few more minutes on a low–medium heat.

Add chopped herbs and stir fry for 10 more minutes on a medium heat.

Add tamarind purée along with half a cup of water and keep on medium low heat for another 15 to 20 minutes.

Gently place fried fish pieces into the sauce. Add salt, pepper and more water if needed. Taste and adjust seasonings. Leave for 30 minutes on low heat. Do not mix or stir after adding fish to the pan.

When ready, plate up and serve with plain long grain basmati rice.

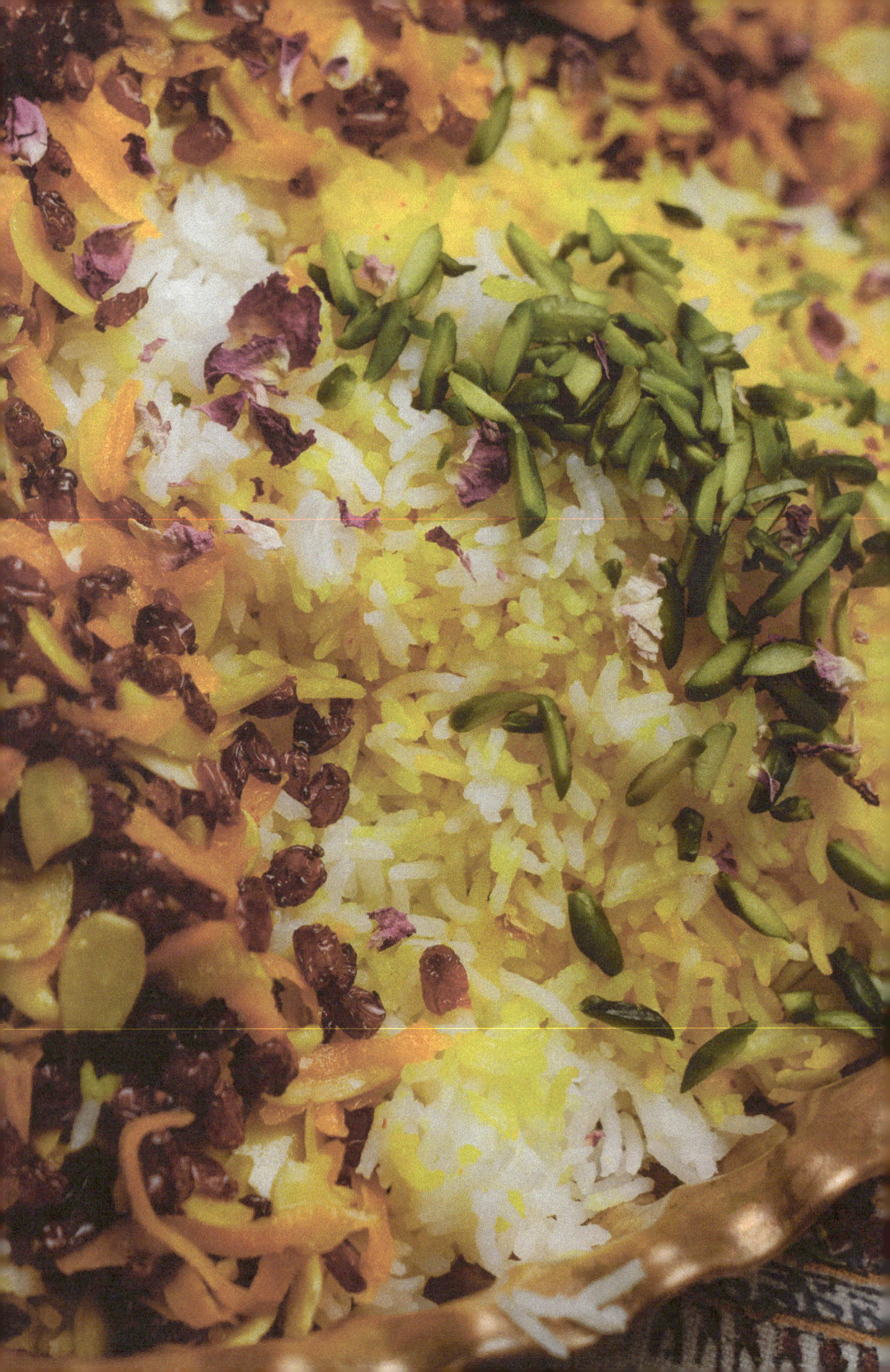

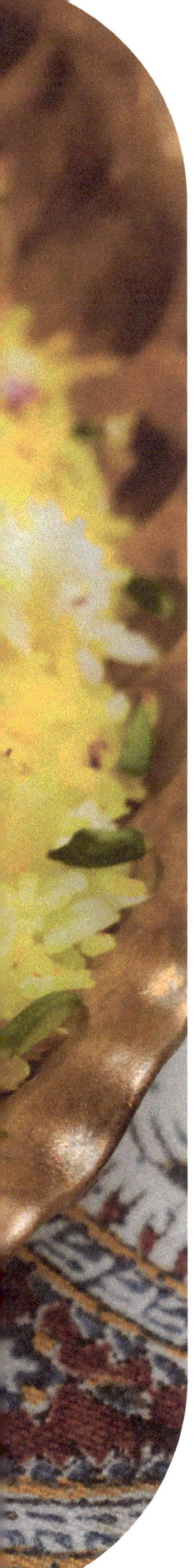

Gheymeh Nesar
(or jewelled rice)

'Ghaymeh' means small pieces of meat and 'Nesar' means generous offering. As the ingredients in this food are all expensive nuts and spices, the person who is offering this food to his guest must be a generous person. All the nuts and colourful barberries on top of this dish makes it look like a jewellery box, so it is also called jewelled rice.

This is the most colourful and famous food from Qazvin province, normally served at weddings and formal religious ceremonies. Qazvin has a long history and was the capital of Iran for 40 years during the Safavi dynasty. In the history of Iran, Qazvin is considered to be the origin for all luxurious food – like pomegranate and rice or pistachio and rice. Some of these foods are not on Iranian menus anymore – even many Iranians have never tried or know much about them – but their presence in Iran's history can't be denied.

Then, there was a lady named Nesa – a very common woman name in those days – who was a single mother. Less common in those days, she ran a catering business to support herself. People used to order her food and by the time for lunch or dinner, would come and collect from her house. Nesa invented Gheymeh Nesar for her richer customers, and whenever they had food as tasty and aromatic as her food elsewhere, to give positive feedback, they would say it tastes and smells like Nesa's food. Nesa was a very thin lady and some people used to call her Nazar (meaning someone who is extremely thin) and they used to call this Gheymeh Nazar. But people didn't like to give this name to the food as it was a shame to give such a name to such a beautiful dish so it returned to being called Gheymeh Nesar again and has been called the same since then. Since rich people used to communicate with court people, the court cook heard about Nesa's food and invited her to work in the court kitchen instead of doing her own catering. This is how this food came to be served to guests of the king.

In those days, nearly 500 years ago, it was not common to eat food with forks and spoons (it was only after the Safavi dynasty, when Iran's borders opened to more travellers and more ambassadors, especially from western countries that people learned more about other styles of eating food, like using forks, spoons and knives). So in formal court gatherings during the Safavi dynasty, food was served on big round copper tray, each for 6 to 7 people. The same food was repeatedly set around each side of the tray so all 6 to 7 people could reach the food. Before serving food, two servants for each group of guests would come around with a big bowl, big jar and clean pieces of towel (one carrying the bowl and jar and the other carrying towel) for them to wash and dry their hands before being served. Sometimes, as a sign of respect, people would use rose water instead of water for guests to wash their hands .

To serve, a large piece of flatbread was left on the bottom tray and then rice, topped with meat, sauce, nuts and spices. Each person around the tray could then start eating from their own side.

At the beginning, the pieces of meat used in this dish were not as small as today, since serving guests with small pieces of meat was a sign of humiliation. After people started learning the western style of eating, with forks and knives, it was hard for people to shred meat with their forks so cooks started to small pieces of meat instead.

Gheymeh Nesar is not usually a normal day-to-day food since it needs a bit of time and effort to prepare. The spices used in this food are heavenly aromatic and to get it to the right place you will need the best quality rice and fresh lamb as well.

Serves 4

Cooking time: 2.5 hours

For meat:

- 300 grams of lamb, ideally lean lamb leg (or chicken – in this case, chicken breast is the best option) cut into small, 3 cm cube pieces
- 2 tbsp vegetable oil
- 1 medium onion, finely chopped
- 1/2 tsp turmeric
- 1 large cinnamon stick
- 1/2 tsp ground cumin
- 1/2 tsp ground cardamom
- 1/4 tsp black pepper
- 3 tbsp tomato purée or one tbsp tomato paste
- Salt as needed

For rice:

- 2 cups long grain basmati rice, washed until the water is clear and soaked with 3 tbsp of salt at least two hours in advance
- 1 piece of Lebanese flatbread or potato, thinly sliced for the bottom of the pot (Tahdig)
- 2 tbsp of vegetable oil (for Tahdig)
- 25 grams butter (for the top of the rice)
- Brewed saffron (to garnish the rice)

For garnish:

- Dried silvered orange peel, soaked in cold water overnight (change the water several times)
- 2 tbsp of sugar
- 2 tbsp of rose water
- 2 tbsp of dried barberries, well washed and drained
- Slivered almonds

- Slivered pistachios
- 30 grams of butter
- 1/3 tsp ground rose pedals

Method

To cook the meat, heat two tablespoons of vegetable oil in a medium pan on a medium heat and add lamb or chicken and chopped onion. and keep, add turmeric, cinnamon stick, cumin, pepper, cardamom and cook for few minutes, stirring occasionally.

Add tomato purée or tomato paste, stir and cook for few more minutes before adding hot boiling water, to cover the meat. Lower the heat, pop the pot lid on and leave to cook until the meat is very soft and until the sauce has thickened. This will take about one hour.

To cook the rice,

Bring a pot (non-stick or Teflon is always the best option for cooking rice) 3/4 filled with water to the boil. When water is boiling, add soaked rice.

When the grains of rice look soft outside and still hard inside, it's time to drain the rice. Gently rinse with warm water without mixing too much. Wash Teflon pot.

Heat two tablespoons of vegetable oil in the Teflon pot. When it looks hot, set flatbread or thin slices of potato to the bottom of the pot. Gradually add the rest of the rice.

Make few holes in the rice to steam the rice.

Push the rice into the shape of a mountain peak and add melted butter on top of the rice. If the rice looks too hard, add one fifth of a cup of water to the top of the rice.

Place the pot over a high heat for five minutes, wrapping the lid with a clean tea towel. After five minutes, cook on a very low heat for at least 45 minutes. Do not remove the lid while the rice is cooking.

After 45 minutes, if the rice around the bottom of the pot looks caramelised, the rice is ready.

Take the rice off the heat with lid and towel still on to keep warm.

To prepare garnishes: drain the orange peel, cook for 10 seconds on a low heat with half a tablespoon of sugar, one tablespoon of oil and 2 tablespoons of rose water. Set aside.

Then cook barberries on a very low heat with one tablespoon of oil and half a tablespoon of sugar for ten seconds.

Put a few spoons of rice in a bowl and add some brewed saffron. Mix and set aside.

To serve, put half of the cooked rice on a plate. Spoon the meat over the rice, then pour the rest of rice on top so the rice is covering the meat. Make into a round shape. Garnish with saffron rice, silvered almonds, silvered pistachios, silvered orange peel and barberries (How you garnish this food depends on how much you care about presentation. You can follow these instructions or you may want to garnish the rice in a more artistic way like you're painting a masterpiece.)

Importantly, like many other Persian foods, this food should be served hot to get the best taste. Iranians have an expression for cold food: they say it's fallen off from your mouth, which means there is no pleasure in eating it.

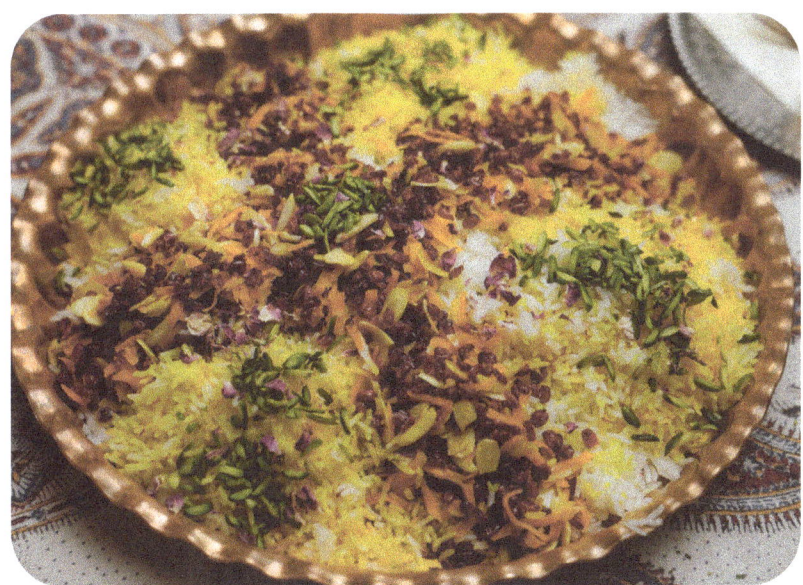

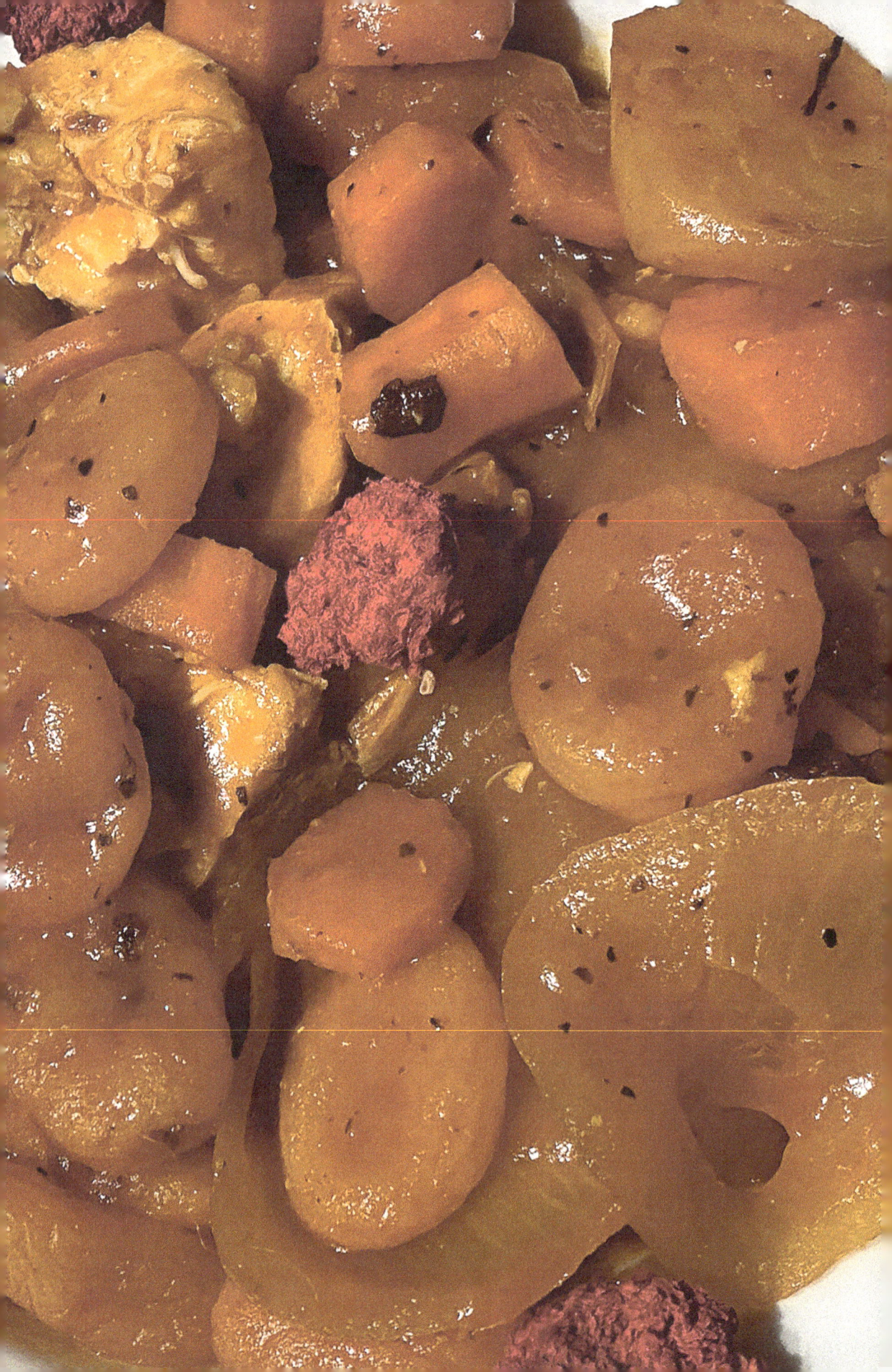

Tas Kabab

Tas is a small copper pot with a specially designed lid – as you put the lid on, it looks the lid is locked to the pot but it can easily be taken off by pushing up the two copper handles on each side.

The quince in this dish gives a subtle, pleasant sweet taste, and Iranians usually use a copper pot to cook quince as they think this allows a good colour to come out of the quince. If quince is cooked in a copper pot, depending on the length of cooking, its yellowish colour will turn from pink, to shiny red.

Originally belonging to the city of Kashan, quince is a very healthy seasonal food that is only available for a few weeks during Autumn. One of closest cities to the capital of Tehran, Kashan is also famous for having the best rose water in the country, the and highest number of traditional houses registered as national heritage. All these houses have been turned into museums now, if you ever visit these houses in Kashan city, you will see quince trees in their big yards.

This food was more common when hunting was very popular among men, including kings. All Iranian kings were very professional at hunting and they were very proud of this talent. There were some special times of the year when the king would go on hunting trips in the jungles with a number of people from the court. Each person had their own tent with as luxurious facilities as could be provided in those days. The king's tent would be in the centre, with all the other tents arranged in a circular shape around his tent. This was also in case of attack – if anyone wanted to get to the king's, tent they had to pass through the other tents and so the residents of those tents could help protect the king.

During this trips, they would normally hunt deer, wild mountain ram and other edible wild animals living in the mountains. Whatever was hunted during the day was sent to the court cook to butcher and use for that night's dinner. In autumn, when there were also a lot of wild fruit trees like quince, Tas Kabab, was one of the first options. The Qajar king used to hunt near Kashan a lot, and maybe this is the reason Tas Kabab originated from this place.

Cooking this dish needs a lot of passion as it has very little water in it. All the juice and water comes from cooking the ingredients on a very low heat. Cooked with very little oil, Tas Kabab is very healthy too.

It's also a dish that needs layering, and you must know which food comes first, otherwise some of the ingredients will easily fall apart and it will lose its shape and consistency. In the original recipe, first layer starts with any edible tree leaves, like vine leaves, but nowadays people usually skip this layer. Different states will use different vegetables in Tas Kabab, but all of them will use quince.

Although it carries the name of Kabab – which is normally given to barbecue or grilled meat – it has no similarities to normal kebabs

Although it has all good ingredients, this comfort food is more for family gatherings, than something you would be served in formal parties. If you are visiting an Iranian person's home for the first time, they would rarely cook this for you unless you ask for it.

You can feel the beautiful blend of spices and enjoy the golden colour of autumn nature in this dish.

Serves 4

Cooking time: 3.5 hours

- 1 tbsp vegetable oil
- 5 medium vine leaves or cabbage leaves for the bottom layer

- 2 large onion
- 1 kg of fatty lamb, or other meat, cut into medium cubes
- 1/2 tbsp turmeric
- 1/2 tsp ground cinnamon
- 1/2 tsp salt
- 1/2 tbsp black pepper
- 2 large carrots, peeled and sliced
- 1 large quince, peeled and sliced (if you can't find quince, replace with hard green apple)
- 2 medium potatoes, peeled and sliced
- 1/2 cup pitted dried prunes
- 1/2 cup tomato purée or 1 tbsp tomato paste
- 2 tbsp fresh lemon juice
- 1 cup water

Method

Pour oil into a pot, preferably a copper pot if you have one.

Set the first layer with flattened vine leaves.

For the second layer, leave big slices of onion.

Season meat with turmeric, cinnamon, salt and pepper.

Set meat on top of the sliced onion.

Layer carrot, quince, tomato, potato and finally, prunes to cover potato.

Sprinkle rest of salt.

Mix tomato paste with lemon juice and water and gently pour all over.

Covered and leave to cook for two and a half hours on a low heat until the meat is tender.

After two and a half hours, if the potato is soft, it's ready to plate up

Food for special religious or national occasions

Although there is a huge amount of advice for food consumption in Muslim culture, the marriage between food and religion was seen during the Safavi dynasty, continuing through the Qajar dynasty until now.

The Safavi dynasty saw a lot of changes in art, culture and food culture. During this time, people started donating special kinds of foods for religious purposes and that's why some special foods are now mainly served on some religious occasions. Some national occasions in the Iranian calendar are also celebrated with certain foods. And some foods started being used in funerals. Whether cooked for religious or national reasons, the cooking processes for these foods carry some interesting common traditions.

These food traditions have a very strong place in people lives. But whether or not people are strongly connected to these traditions, it seems to impossible to separate these foods from their traditional roots.

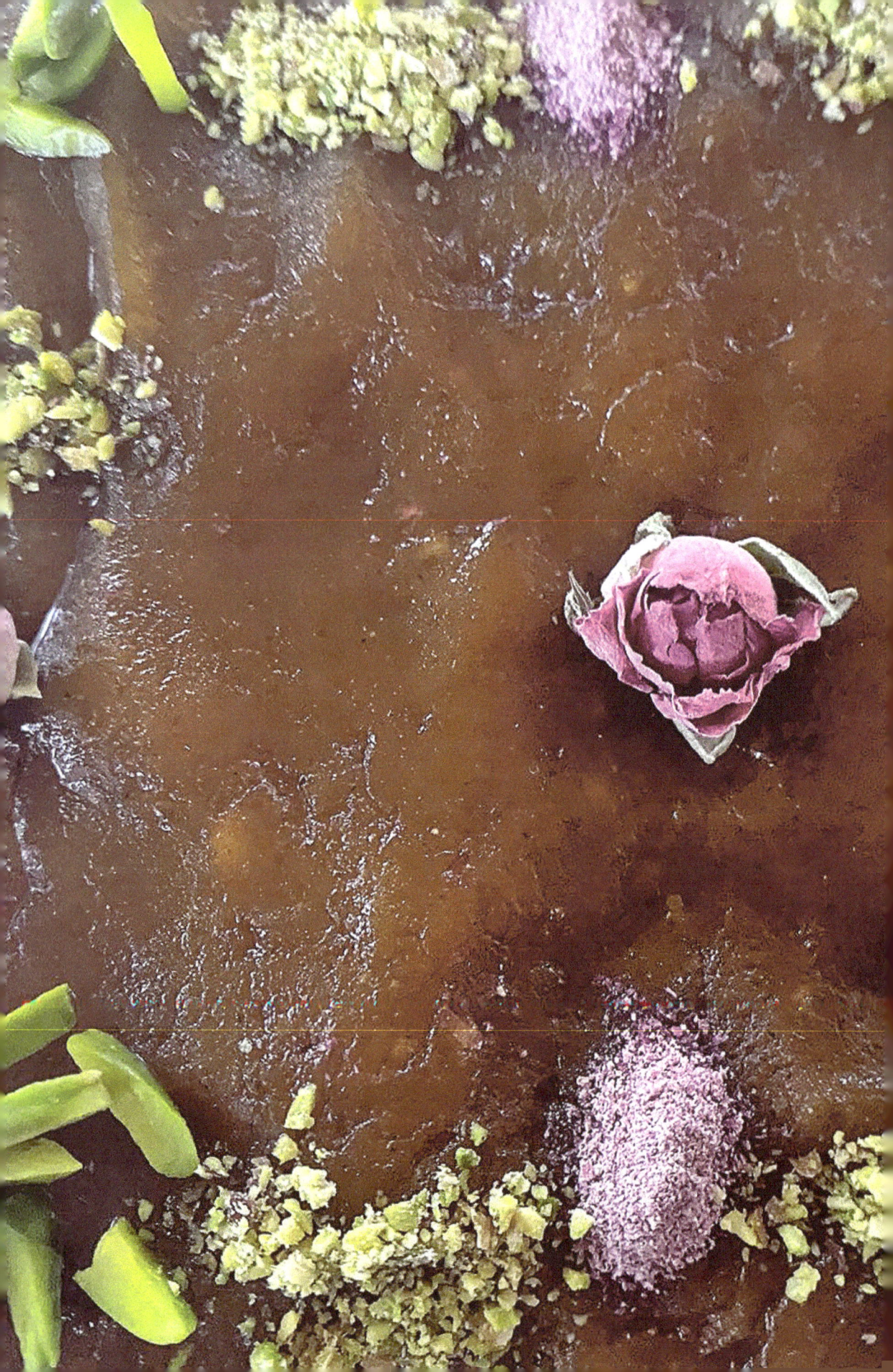

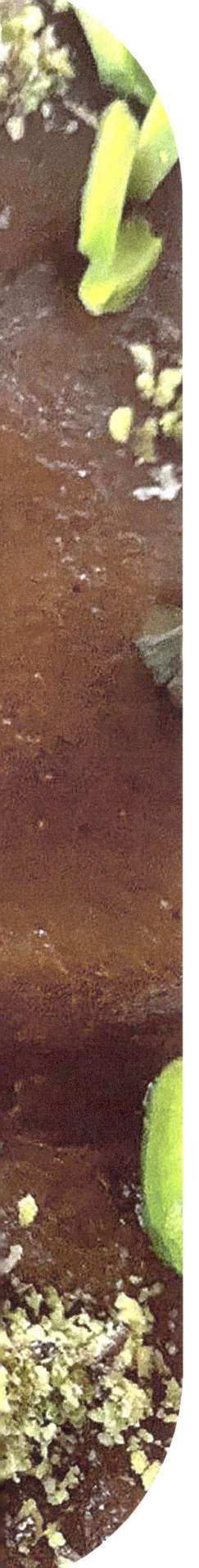

Halva

Halva is a sweet dense paste made of flour, butter, sugar syrup, saffron, rose water and cardamon powder. It's said to originally be an Arab dessert but its taste and easy preparation meant it made its way to many other countries, including Iran. Persian Halva is completely different from other kinds of Halva. in Iran. Halva is a constant food in every funeral, later generations believed the scent and aroma comes from Halva while it's being cooked comes from heaven and for this reason it makes devil run away from that funeral.

Halva's hero ingredient is wheat flour. Wheat has a very special place in Iranian historic myths. There are a large number of poems and stories about respecting grain like wheat, and in mythic stories its origin is straight from heaven. But mainly, these stories come from a time when agriculture was not mechanised. Bread was always a dominant daily product, but it was a hard and time consuming process make flour out of grain. So, wheat and its products became considered object to respect, since it was people's staple food. Even these days, if older people find a piece of bread on the street they kiss it and put it in their eyes – which means it's as dear to you as your eyes – and then leave it somewhere where people can't step on it. They believed even a piece of leftover bread in the street might be used by a hungry homeless person, so it shouldn't be left where people can walk on it.

Like every other Persian food there is huge variety of Halva. Every state has their own recipe, but some ingredients like flour, sugar and saffron are main ingredients in all those recipes. Here, I give you the most common recipe, which is the one that is served to guests at funerals and memorial services.

This recipe uses clarified butter mixed with flour giving which a mix of plant and animal products. In traditional beliefs, Halva is a food which brings unity between two essences and worlds of plants and animals.

Serves 4

Cooking time: 1 hour

- 1/2 cup butter
- 1 cup wheat flour
- 2–3 tbsp vegetable oil
- 1 cup sugar
- 2 cups water
- 1/2 cup rose water
- 1/2 tsp saffron, brewed or dissolved in 3 tbsp of boiling water
- 1/2 tbsp ground cardamom

Method

Heat butter in a medium pan over a medium heat. Once butter is melted, add flour and put on a very low heat.

Stir continuously and passionately until the flour changes to golden brown in colour. If needed, add 2 to 3 tablespoons of vegetable oil and mix well. Set aside

Mix water and sugar over a medium heat, stirring every now and then. When the liquid starts to thicken into a syrup, add rose water, saffron and cardamom.

Stir syrup well and gently, gradually add to your mix of golden brown flour (do not pour syrup to flour at once).

Put the saucepan back onto a medium heat and stir continuously. After 5 minutes, turn down to a low heat and continue to stir until the mixture thickens.

When the mixture is thick, take off the heat and let it cool down.

Spread the mixture flat on a plate and garnish with any desired nuts, ideally slivered almonds and pistachios, with rose petals

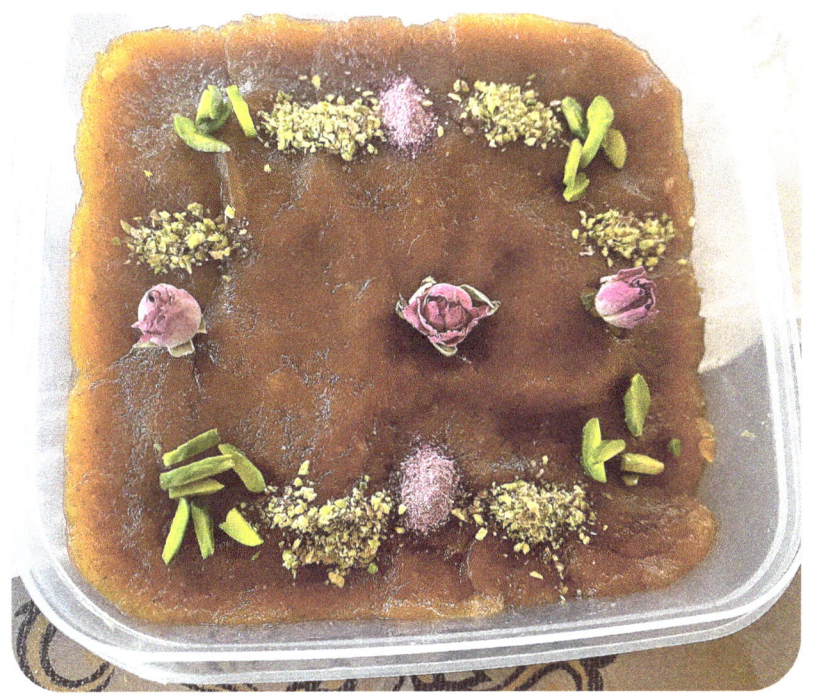

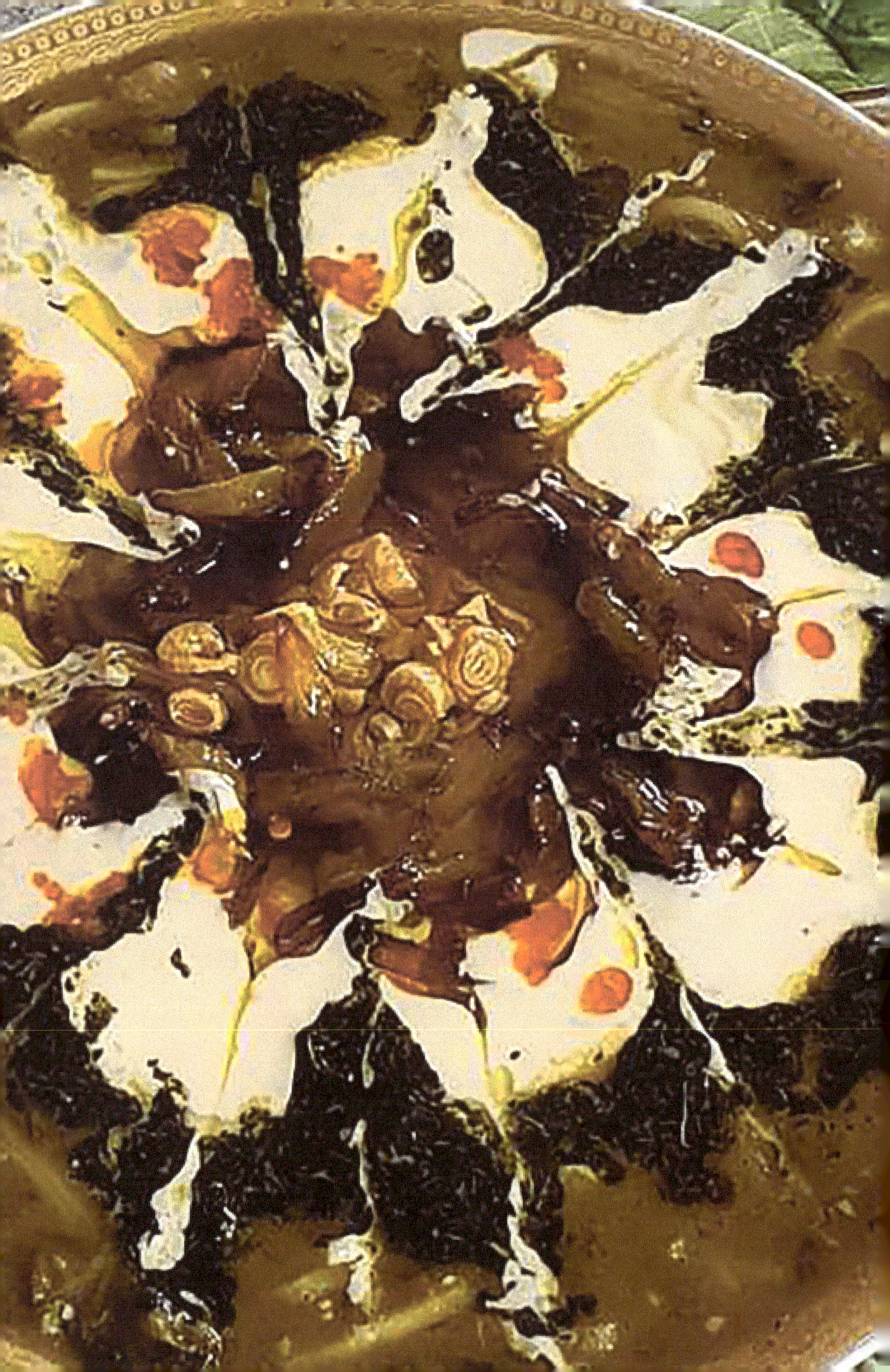

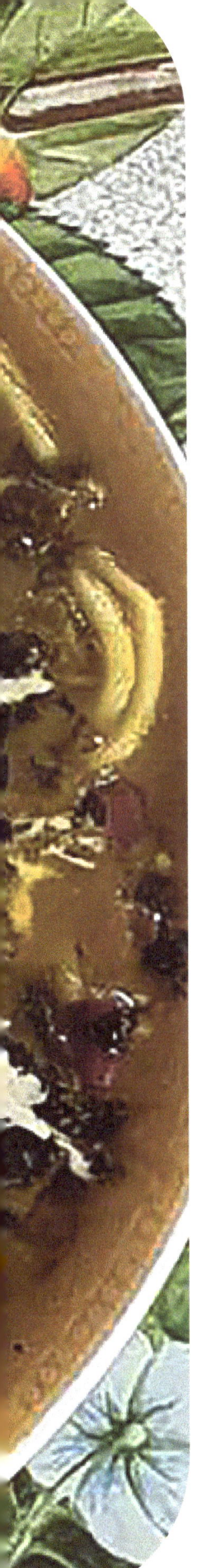

Ash-E-Shoo-Le-Ghalam Kar

There is very famous proverb among Iranian whenever they face with someone or some situations very disorganised they say it looks like Ash-e- Shoo-Le- Ghalam Kar.

Since in this particular Ash you can find all sorts of beans, every kind of grains and herbs and there is no special order for most of its ingredients, which means all sorts of beans and herbs could be used in it.

That's why people brought it in to a proverb to prove something disorganised but not messy.

Yet there is another common proverb among people about this Ash. When someone is complaining about a job seems hard to them but not very hard actually, people answer them back what's so complain about? Your not cooking Ash - E- Shoo- le- Ghalamkar which points how hard and how time consuming is processing this food.

Yet both and later proverbs about this Ash proves how seriously people took cooking this Ash.

Although it has a very long and historic background, it just started being very popular among people as a Nazri food and especially in religious ceremonies nearly 150 years ago.

Here is the story :

Nearly 150 years ago there was a sudden Cholera breakdown in Tehran capital city where was residency for King and his court people. Many people had died, even King Nasser - Al-Din- Shah was contracted by Cholera very seriously. He was so sick everyone in court though he is not going to survive. His special chef in court cooked him this Ash and Shah had it after long time not being able to eat. He found it very tasty and day after he had this Ash with almost everything in it, he felt much better.

A few weeks after when he totally felt well, he decided to distribute this Ash as Nazri among people in early days of each spring. The most strange part of his Nazri was he said he was personally is going to help in cooking this Ash and work like his servants. Everyone was so surprised as everyone in court knew how lazy he was, he had never done hard work in his life and had now decided to work in the preparation of this Ash like a servant under supervision of the highest chef in the court. That means when King is going to be working all people of the court must follow the job or they are going to be in trouble.

He chose one of his palace gardens for cooking the Ash and asked for 13 huge, giant big pots,with actual firewood for cooking in garden.

Chef also ordered the pots to be set in one line on cooking day. No one in court was ever brave enough to disagree with Shah, so everyone in court not only agreed with his decision, but also praised it as the best decision Shah ever made, they also said they all are ready to work lik servants that day to help the King to accomplish his Nazri. All minsters and princes and princess es were working that day cleaning, washing, peeling and frying.

The King also asked for the best quality ingredients to be in the Ash so he asked his special chef to prepare the best quality ingredients and ask for help from his court people in every step of cooking Ash. The King as I said was a lazy man and no one had ever seen him doing even his own personal jobs, he announced infront of everyone, he is going to work like a servant that day. But in reality the only thing he did was sit on top of a well decorated bed in the garden infront of the pots which were set in a long line and started smoking, with all others gathering around him, infront of each of the big trays of ingredients the court people started cleaning and preparing ingredients under supervision of the court chef. Each one of them were trying to pretend they are working harder than others infront of Shah to make him believe how loyal they are to Shah and his Nazri .

But his court people were also as lazy as the King and working hard infront of Shah was a big day for those men and women who had never got their hands dirty in their life.

This was a funny show because secretly all court kitchen hands were doing all the work and the court people were only pretending to work very hard infront of Shah. Each one we're secretly trying to somehow screw others and put heavy duties on their shoulders. At the end of the day this bunch of lazy yet flattery people who have never worked hard in their life were so exhumed even though in reality they didn't do much work anyway. The whole day they were involved somehow and that was such heavy job for them. For this Ash takes almost a whole day get to the right point to be ready to eat.

It needs to be cooked on low heat on firewood and stirred constantly otherwise it will burn easily and that won't give the pleasant taste to the Ash. This means it's very time consuming process and it won't be ready until next day. By late afternoon that day all court people went back to their homes while all the servants continued on cooking and stirring process especially during the night as it was crucial to keep on stirring until the next morning after sunrise. By then it should be ready .

The next day early morning the Ash was ready and court special chef would send a bowl to each one of court people to have it as breakfast. Still many people believe it's best to have this Ash as breakfast. Sending a bowl of this Ash to court people house was the beginning of another proverb and story which still people use in some situations.

When chefs sent bowl of Ash to each one court people they were supposed to fill it with gold and return it back to King as a sign of how happy they were that their King survived from illness. Also they could prove they were giving their gold to charity to Thank God bringing back health to their King.

They knew the bigger would be the bowl, the more they had to fill it with gold by the time of returning the bowl to the chef. Still in Iran if a neighbour or friend brings you a plate of any kind of food Iranian have this tradition to never return the plate empty, there is always something as sign for thanking the sender. Each one of court people asked chef secretary to send them small bowl of Ash instead they would do favours for chef during the whole year. This made the court chef very powerful man in the court almost all minster and princes were scared of him. During whole year if chef asked them a favour and if court people wouldn't or couldn't accomplish his favour, on Nazri day chef would send them really a big bowl. For those who really couldn't afford sending bowl back full of gold needed to borrow gold and then send it back to court .

Later people made this proverb popular among people on behalf of the chef: Ok you don't do me a favour I know what kind of Ash to cook you when the day comes, I cook a big bowl of Ash with lots of oil on top and that meant on Nazri day he is going to send them a big bowl of Ash which should be returned back full of gold otherwise King would be cross with them. Still when someone is so upset with others they want to put a threat on them they say: When time comes I know what kind of Ash to cook you, I will cook you a Ash with lots of oil on top and that means your gonna be in trouble when time comes.

But that's not the only proverb generated particularly by this food, there is also another very famous proverb among people which still are both very commonly used. And I really mean both just start getting popular after King Nazri. As I said above in a day of cooking, Nazri King and his court people pretended to work hard. Everyone else was trying but the court people only pretended infront of the King.

Also as I said they all were princess and minsters from highest level of society who never worked in their life so it was so strange for labourers watching them working, some where frying eggplants which is very time consuming and needs patience to get the right colour. But as they wanted to pleased the King so they were frying eggplants very precisely for later garnishing of the Ash bowl (eggplant is not in the actual recipe it was just the che'sf idea for garnish), this was a source for a proverb to anyone who was apple shinning, and flattering others, others say: look he is garnishing plates with eggplant – which refers to that person's flattering attitude.

Serving: 8

Preap : 2 hours

Time: 2-4 hours best result comes on very low heat cooking

- All sorts of beans could be used in this Ash except green beans
- 1/4 cup from each kind of beans washed and soaked over night
- 1/4 cup green lentil (always cook green lentil separately and then add to Ash later)
- 1/4 cup chickpeas washed and soaked over night

- 1 large onion, peeled and cut in 4 for cooking with meat
- 1 median cup of rice
- 2 pounds beef ribs
- 2 tablespoons turmeric
- 4 large onion, chopped finely fried to crisp, add later to Ash.
- Herbs: Dill, parsley, coriander, chives, spinach, 2 bunch of each, washed, well chopped.
- 1/4 cup washed, well chopped fresh tarragon or two tablespoons of dried tarragon

Flavour of tarragon in this Ash is very important, it's the flavour of tarragon and black pepper which gives distinguished taste to this Ash compared to other sorts of Ash.

- Salt as desired

Black pepper (as said above flavour of black pepper should be more dominantly tasted in this Ash compared to others and it must be black pepper not because of the heat but it's flavour since the flavour for black pepper is different from chilli but no exact amount is given because it depends how strong you like this flavour in your food)

For garnish:

- 2 large onion, thin sliced and fried in 3 tablespoons of vegetable oil to golden crisp
- 4 cloves of garlic thinly sliced and fried in two tablespoons of vegetable oil to golden to crisp
- 2 tablespoons of dried mint fried in oil with 1 teaspoon of turmeric for only 20 seconds

Method

Place all beans soaked overnight in a big bowl, add enough water to cover top of the beans. Leave on low heat until soft. Add lentil in another smaller bowl with same way and cook with water until it's soft but not very soft, green lentil shouldn't be cooked with beans as lentil cooks faster than beans.

Once all cooked, mix cooked beans with cooked lentil and set them aside.

In another pot add rice with 3-4 cups of water and leave on medium low heat until rice are very soft and mushy during cooking if rice water was all gone add another cup of water to rice pot.

Then add cooked rice to beans and lentils which are already cooked. Leave on medium low heat and give occasional stir and then add all chopped herbs and continue on giving occasional stir until herbs colour is changed to dark and they're soft too.

In another pot add beef tubes with 4 quartered onion and 1 teaspoon of turmeric, water should be cover the ribs and leave for 45 min-1 hours until meat is soft and well cooked. Once meat in ribs are well cooked and it's soft and tender time to take them out of broth and finely shredded the meat.

Meat must be falling off from the bones so you can easily be able to shred it.

Add broth with 2/3 of shredded meat to all other cooked ingredients and leave 1/3 of shredded meat for garnish later.

In large fry pan add 4 tablespoons of vegetable oil and fry thinly sliced onion for 15-20 min on medium low heat until sliced onions turn to crispy.

Add 2/3 fried onion to the pot mixture and leave the rest for garnish later.

Stir all ingredients in the pot occasionally to stop it from burning while you start frying sliced garlic in another smaller pan with 3 tablespoons of vegetable oil.

Once garlic colour was slightly changed add 2/3 to the big pot mixture and leave 1/3 for garnish later.

In another smaller pan add 3 tablespoons of vegetable oil and dried mint with 1/2 tablespoons of turmeric and just fry for not more than 20 minutes otherwise it will burn and colour and taste both will be unpleasant.

Meanwhile frying onions, garlic and mint occasionally give a stir to the big pot mixtures.

Time to add black pepper and salt, remember black pepper should be tasted well in every spoon but not give a super hot taste to the Ash, just feeling dominant flavour is enough.

Leave all cooked ingredients on very low heat for 45 more minutes, do not stop giving occasional stir.

Now your Ash is ready to plate up in any small or big bowl you want.

For topping you can add Kashk (earlier I described what is Kashk in other recipes) or even Greek yogurt but it's not a must to have it with Kashk or yogurt, it's delicious enough even without these two.

Use left shredded meat and fried onion and garlic and fried mint for garnish.

I suggest having it in a very cold or rainy morning as breakfast and Noosh E Jan

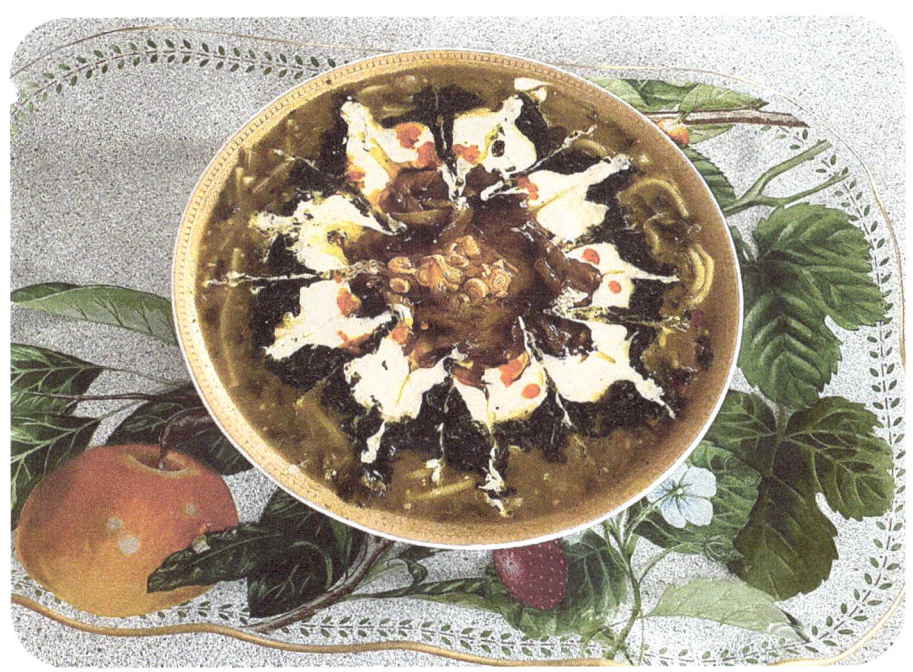

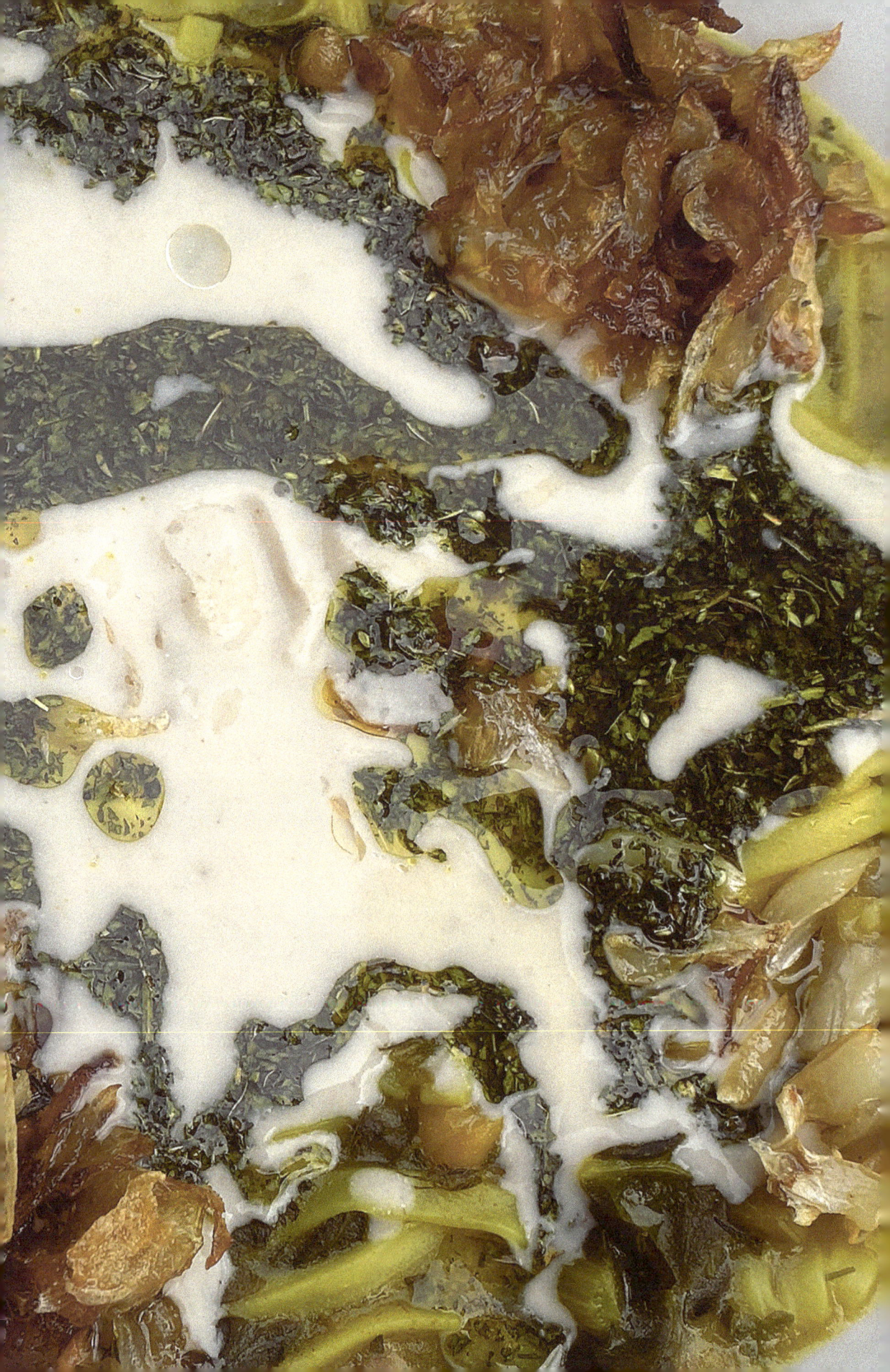

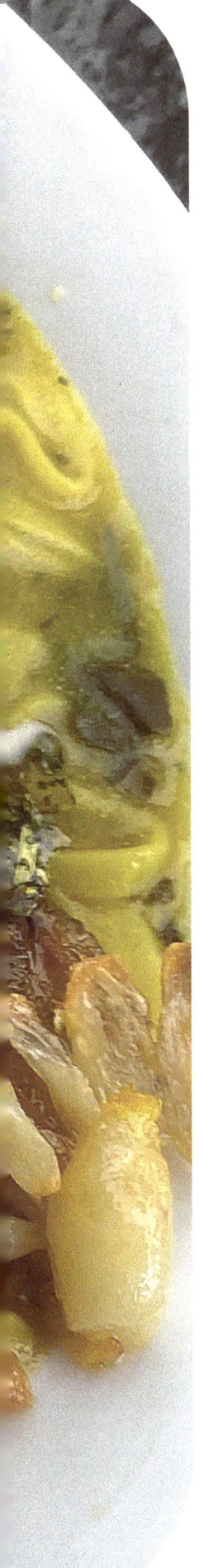

Ash-e-Ash-E-Reshteh (Persian nodule soup)

Ash- e - reshteh is a traditional Persian noodles soup.

In Iranian food culture Ash (or persian soup) has very special place .

For this recipe I really didn't know wether I should mention it in food for special occasions or write in another section as seasonal section but very well fits both and very popular in both situations.

Cooking in persian in word is called (Ash- Pazi=Ash=soup and Pazi=cooking). Word Ash is in the first syllable of this task in defining cooking process which proves for Iranian in old days cooking process was mostly about producing Ash in the kitchen.

I really wasn't sure in which section I should fit Ash-e-Reshteh, whether it should be in seasonal food or it should fit in food for special occasions as it could perfectly fit both.

It's hard to say which ingredients in this dish is having the honour to be the hero ingredient as they all have a key role in producing good Ash.

A good Ash comes out of lots of beans in fact all sorts of beans could be used in Ash which means feel free to use any kind of beans in your Ash except green beans. Lots of herbs, fried onion, fried garlic and fried mint along with Persian white noodles made of wheat flour should be used too.

This combination of all this together makes a very aromatic, amazingly delicious and very nutritious soup.

As I said above all sorts of soup in Persian food vocabulary used to be called Ash except some western style soup recipes which came to Persian food menus nearly 60 years ago after world war ll. They are called soup but before that Persians only had Ash and hardly anyone knew what soup was.

For you, both could be called soup, but for us, Ash has its traditional texture and traditional process to bring it out in the dish and soup is made with some ingredients which we hardly used to have in our Ash.

As I said before nearly 60-70 years ago soup for Iranians was only interpreted to a wide range of Ash and each state had their own signature Ash but among all those Ash the one with noodles was and still is the queen of all sorts of Ash.

Western style food and also soup came to Iranian food menu later when capital city Tehran and later some other states in country were occupied by union forces during world war ll.

Although people didn't like the situation but this historical event had a big impact on their traditions and culture and specially in their eating and cooking style.

Foreign Soldiers introduced lots of new food and recipes to Iranian and later people from first class in society who had chance to travel to overseas also introduced new western style recipes to Iranian daily food menu.

But even with these new attractive foods such as all sorts of soups, Ragout, Gigot, and many years later hamburgers, pizza still didn't cost a bite from their advocacy for traditional food.

To make you understand better about the difference between Ash and soup, I must say for Ash it is a Persian lose dish like soup but most of the time cooked with lots of herbs and beans. It is only few recipes for Ash which there are no herbs or beans in them.

Herbs for all sorts of Ash usually depends on the area it's cooked which usually people use local grown wild herbs. But most of the time main herbs are parsley, coriander, chives and spinach.

There are thousands recipes for Ash as each state have their own signature Ash according to their availability for ingredients.

As different climates all over Iran does not give chance for availability and accessibility to all sorts of ingredients.

Among all these sorts of Ash (Ash -e- reshteh) is the most famous and common one all over the country. It's looks like there is not such long and old history for Ash -e- reshteh as there is not any information about this soup in very old history book. What we know is it's looks like it first was used by people in Turkey and then residents of Azerbaijan and finally Iranian added it to their cuisine list .

The noodles for this soup used to be prepared by hand in each house by themselves made from wheat flour mixed with water and salt. They used to prepare the dough and then cut the nodules in very thin rope shape in length and dry and hanging these rope shape noodles on the lines in sun to be dried and used in winter time.

Today there are commercial version of noodles made in factories easily and like everything else people enjoy of easy version of this ingredient saving their time for more important things in life.

There are some other recipes to cook these noodles soup with adding some extra ingredients but none had been able to compete with this traditional version of Ash -e- Reshteh. Combinations of herbs, fried onion and fried garlic with cooked beans and white noodles all together with topping of a special kind of processed yogurt called Kashk makes everyone to fall in love with this soup.

If you travel in cold seasons to Iran there are some food shops in middle of traditional market they only serve Ash - e- Reshteh during winter and in hot seasons they change their selling products to traditional Persian drinks like saffron cold drink.

Imagine you are walking in a very traditional Persian market, it's a very cold snowy day in winter, and you can see big pots full of Ash with steam and aroma of fried garlic and mint that comes from it, a seller who invites you with his loud voice singing come, come and eat Ash in a very rhythmic voice and while he is singing he's stirring the Ash with his giant size ladle. It is a very interesting scene for every visitors who likes to know about Iran more that you should see for yourself.

In many traditional national or religions ceremonies different sorts of Ash and mainly this noodles Ash is served as Nazri which I have described earlier Ash is also very common in Nazri food list.

For best result and to boost the taste and flavour they sometimes add lamb or beef. Once the bone is cooked and flavour of broth is there, they take out the bones and throw it since bone itself doesn't have give nice appearance to the Ash, then other ingredients will be added to the pot one by one. Ash -e- reshteh specially is one of those food you need to know lots of hacks to get to the right point.

Not very long from today almost 150 years ago Ash and Abgoosht were dominantly on people cooked menu for their daily food. Even for rich people and for court people it didn't matter how many fantasy and luxurious food swas served Ash and mainly Ash with noodles was always on the table specially in very cold days.

Of course those days only rare people from very high social status used to sit and eat around a table. Others used to gather and sit around a what we call a table cover mainly made of hand painted fabric which is a handicraft from historical city Isfahan, back then there was no plastic table cover.

Food served in normal people house was usually very simple, those who could afford in cold season had either Ash or Abgoosht for cold season specially for rainy and snowy days and for hot season they usually had either cold yogurt soup or fresh fruit which was usually watermelon or honeymoon with cheese and bread. For those who were so poor couldn't afford cooked food, it was usually bread and cheese with sweetened tea in cold days and bread and yogurt in hot days.

It might be hard to believe but during World War ll for most of the people daily food was limited to only bread and in many cases they didn't even have bread and used to eat whatever vegetable they could grow in their backyard. Very hard days were those days, thousands of people all around the country died of hunger. Anyway back to our beloved Ash -e- Reshteh as you can understand it is definitely a seasonal food but it's popularity doesn't not let this food to be limited only for cold days, sometimes Ash lovers cook it even in a middle of summery hot days, Of course having it on a very cold rainy days is something else.

Farmers in western states where weather is very cold sometimes even in summer used to have Ash as breakfast but it was not a very early breakfast, it was a brunch. They used to go to farm very early morning and still go very early to work after they had their morning praying before sunrise.

As I said they go to farm very early before sunrise and because of that they usually don't have a decent breakfast only a tea and later in mid day women take big pots of Ash with themselves to farm and feed their tired men with all sorts of Ash, if it's Ash-e- reshteh they cook its alot lighter than usual with less beans so they won't be too full and can have lunch later too.

They add some diluted thin yogurt to this soup to give more taste but usually processed yogurt which is called Kashk is always served on top of Ash -e-reshteh to add to its taste. It's hard to describe what is Kashk and how does it taste. It made from diluted yogurt with water and boiled until it's get thick, meanwhile they add salt to preserve it too. It's taste is much stronger than yogurt and it's used in many different food and mainly used in different kinds of Ash. But for Ash-e- Reshteh you really don't get the taste if you skip the Kashk. Kashk comes on top of the serving bowl and not in the pot as they said Kashk will lose its flavour if boiled in the pot so it's usually comes to garnish by the time of serving.

Serve : 4-6

Prep time : 2 hours

Cook time : 1 hours

- 1/4 cup of chickpeas,
- 1/4 beans (any kind of dry beans will do mainly red kidney beans or white beans)
- 1/4 cooked green lentil
- 3 large onion thinly sliced
- 5 clove of garlic thinly chopped
- 1 table spoon of dried mint
- 1 tablespoons of turmeric
- 3 cups of stock
- 2 bunch of parsley
- 2 bunch of coriander
- 1 bunch of chives
- 2 bunch of spinach, all washed, drained to take extra water out and very well chopped

- 1 table spoon of all purpose flour
- 1/4 pack wheat Chinese noodles (make sure it's wheat noodles, other kinds of noodles are not very well fitted for this soup).
- 1 large jar of water

Method

Ideally for topping, its better to use Persian processed yogurt called Kashk which could be find in any Persian shop if not available just add Greek yogurt on top by the Tim's of serving.

- 1 cup of Vegetable oil
- Salt and pepper as desired

In a medium size pan add two tablespoons of vegetable oil and fry slices of chopped onion, once onions are golden brown take out and set aside. Again in same pan add oil on medium heat and add sliced garlic and fry till you get light golden colour and set aside.

Cook beans that you have soaked overnight remember to throw the water it's soaked with and add fresh water for cooking beans to the pot. And in medium pot cook beans together.

Cook green lentil in separate pot, and once beans and lentil in separate pot got soft texture it's time to turn off the heat. Transfer cooked beans to another bigger pot and add well chopped herbs, 1/2 turmeric, salt and pepper and bone stock if you use for boosting flavour,and cooked lentil and let them all cook together again until herbs are cooked with beans and broth and colour of herbs changed.

Add 1/2 of fried onion and half 1/2 of fried garlic.

Break the noodles in half and add to the soup.

Once noodles are cooked well in soup, add 1 tablespoon of flour in small cup with cold water, mix well and add to the soup let the mixture combine and cook in the soup, store the soup and once you got a well not so loose texture of soup it's time to turn off the heat. Leave the lid on pot and wait for 10-15 minutes before serving.

Start plating in any preferred bowls and, wait for few minutes and add fried onion and fried garlic on top of each bowl and now add Kashk if you have or 1 tablespoons of Greek yogurt on top of each bowl for garnish.

In a small pan add two tablespoons of vegetable oil and add dry mint powder with left turmeric do not leave on heat for long only 15 seconds in enough, for leaving dry mint on heat for a long time will cause mint powder burn and turn an unpleasant dark colour beside it gives a bitter taste to mints powder.

Add this fried dry mint powder on top of the Ash for garnish and Noosh E Jan.

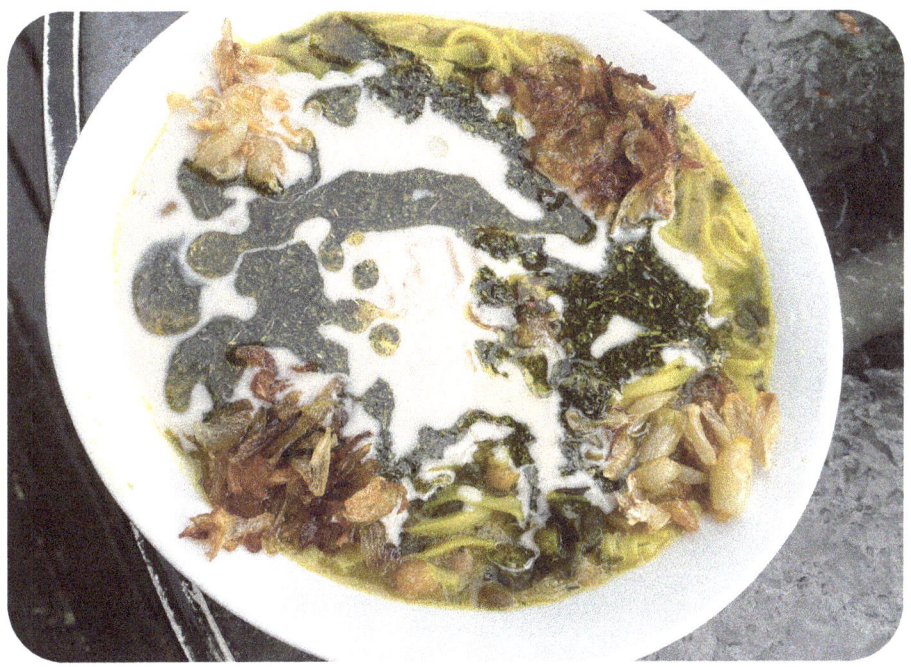

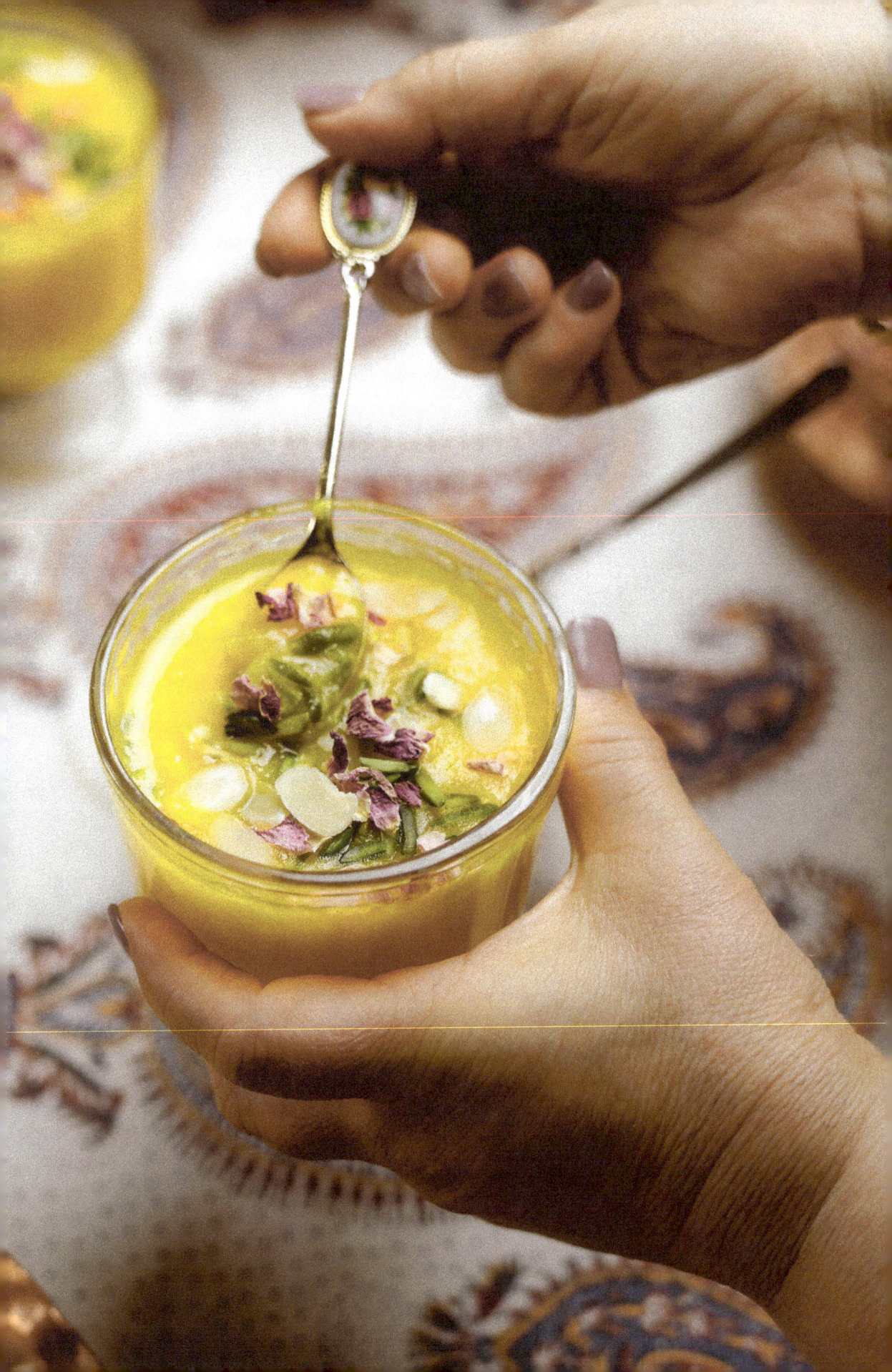

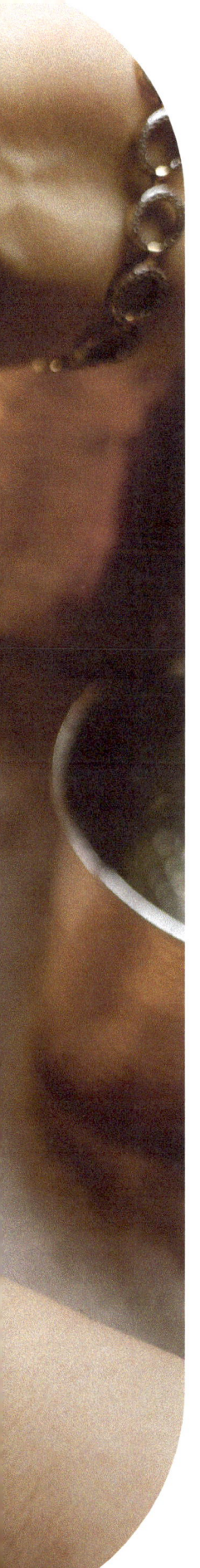

Shoo Le Zard
(saffron rice pudding)

Shoo Le are foods with loose texture, like soups. In Iran, there is a variety of Shoo Le, most of which are originally from either the state of Khoorasan in the north east or from Kermanshah in the west. With its religious reputation, Khoorasan known for stronger in serving foods with religious backgrounds and for religious purposes. Of all the Shoo Le, Shoo Le Zard is sweet and the most famous among them.

In the past, when people mostly used to be poor, richer people used to choose special days of the year – mainly religious days – to give away free food to the poor. There are certain dishes that were more popular to distribute than others on such occasions: Halva, which we already talked about, and Shoo Le Zard were the favourites. But while it is often made in large amounts and widely distributed, that doesn't mean people don't cook it in smaller amounts for their families.

There are some other traditional acts happening while people cook Shoo Le Zard

If it is cooked for a religious ceremony for donations, people might ask others, like friends and family members to come and help, since usually large amounts are cooked and distributed to community members – whether neighbours or just people passing by in the street. This might seem strange to you, to be walking in the street and out of the blue someone offers you a bowl of food, and you might not feel safe eating it, but in Iran, this is a normal scene – especially during a month of religious activities or fasting.

On the donation day, people put big, mostly copper, pots on the streets. Sometimes, if they are cooking very large amounts, maybe feeding more than 100 people, they will they clear the area in advance and lay out stands for giant cooktops. No one stops them from doing this since everyone thinks this is an action for God and his prophets, and stopping these kinds of activities is a big sin that will be punished by God. Everybody helps in these activities – even people you don't know at all will offer help without even being asked.

When the ingredients are cooking on the pot, it needs lots of stirring, normally using extremely big wooden spoons. If you are not strong enough to stir with the big spoon, someone will help you to hold the big spoon. They will be stirring while you just pretend you're stirring, making a wish or praying while you are both stirring together.

Some people will pray around the big pot while the Shoo Le Zard is cooking. When the cooking is finished, they turn the heat off, put the pot lid back and leave it to cool down. After it has cooled, they open the lid to start garnishing and start distributing, and someone is chosen to look at the surface.

Usually, there will be some random design on the surface. People believe these designs could be read as holy words or names of their holy prophets, which they take it as a sign that their wishes and prayers are accepted by God. To garnish, cinnamon powder is used to write holy words or prophets' names on the surface of bowls in which they are serving the food. The second part of the garnish is slivered almonds or pistachios on surface to make it prettier and more desirable.

When all designed and garnished bowls of Shoo Le Zard are distributed ,it's time for those that have participated in the working bee to start eating. Usually, the owner of the process cooks something else for the crew as lunch or dinner. They will throw a large linen, mostly made of nylon, on the floor and leave food in it and all the crew sits around and eats together. Once they have finished eating, everyone will clean up together and wash all dishes and pots. After cleaning, everybody goes home. Sometimes, they won't see each other again until next similar activity.

Serves 4 people
Cooking time: 1 hour

- 1 cup rice, rinsed and soaked in cold water overnight
- 2 cups sugar
- 8 cups water (per 1 cup of rice)
- 1/3 cup butter
- 2 tsp of saffron
- 1/2 cup rose water
- 1/2 cup slivered almonds
- 1/2 tsp ground cardamom
- 1/3 tsp ground cinnamon
- 1 tbsp slivered pistachios
- Rose petals

Method

Drain the rice and place in a large pot along with 8 cups of water. Bring to a boil over a medium heat. When it starts to boil, reduce the heat and let the rice cook until it's soft. If the water has reduced and the rice has not yet fully soft, add more water and keep cooking on low heat, stirring occasionally.

When the water has reduced significantly and the rice is completely soft, add sugar. Cook until the sugar is completely dissolved and water is reduced enough (to about one cup of water). Make sure to keep stirring to prevent the rice from sticking to the bottom of the pot.

Add 3 tablespoons of boiling water to powdered saffron and brew it until the colour changes to a strong orange.

Add butter, cardamom, rose water and brewed saffron and half of the almonds to the pot and stir until most of the number of water has evaporated and the mixture is medium thick.

Turn off the heat and leave the pot until it's cool.

Pour into serving dishes and garnish with the rest of the almonds, pistachios and cinnamon powder, and a few rose petals if you like.

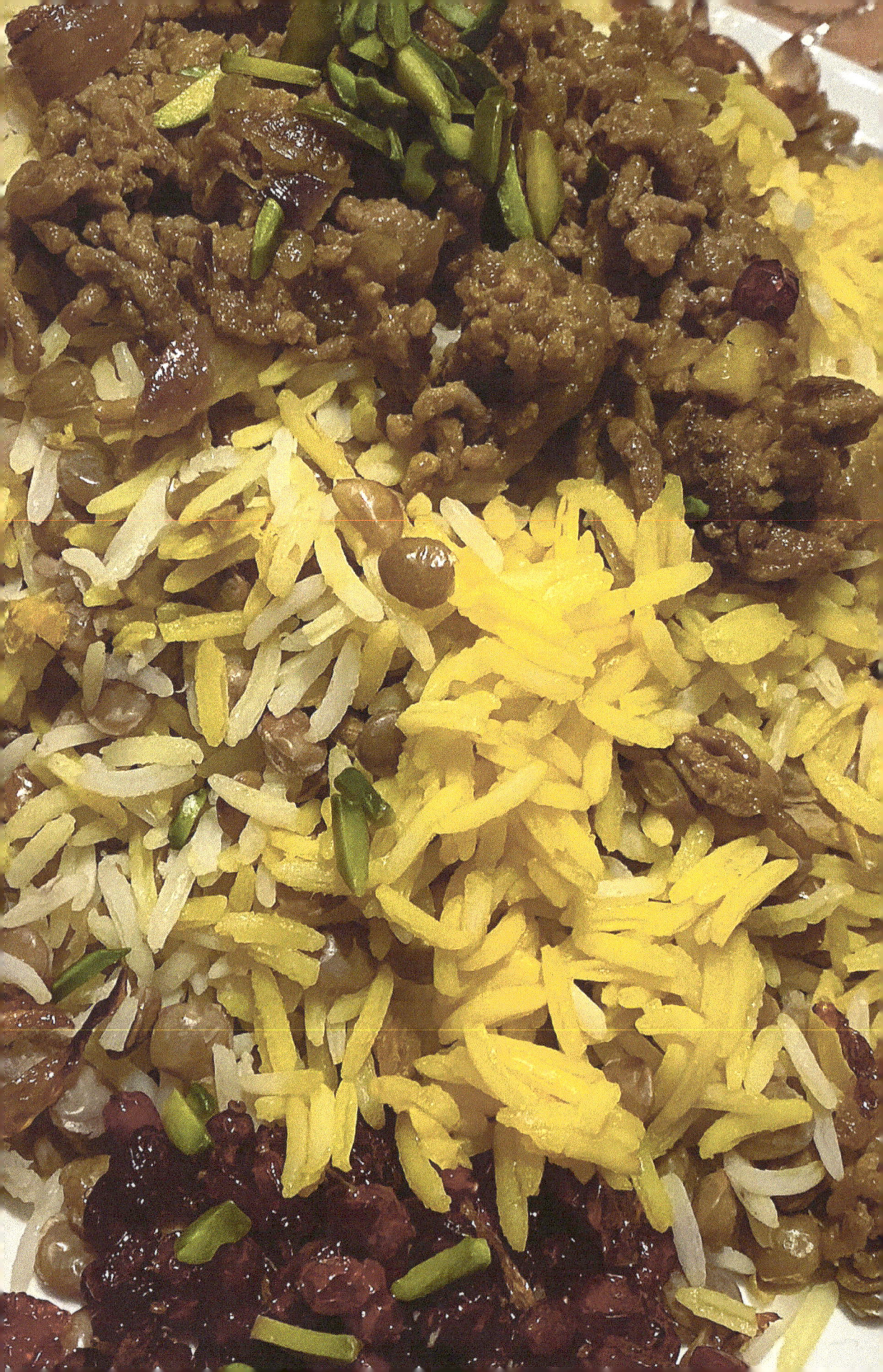

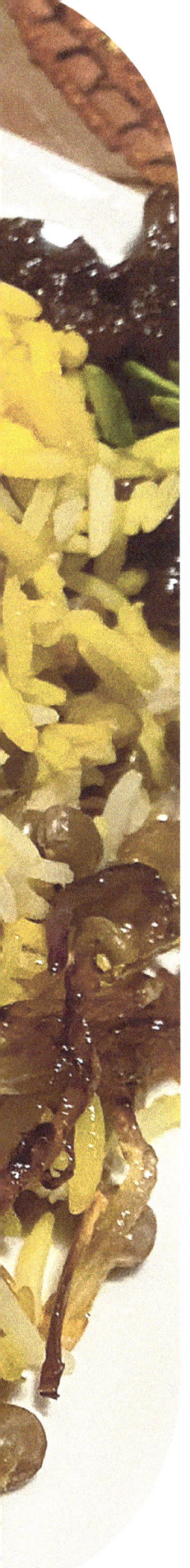

Adas polo
(green lentils and rice with minced meat and raisins)

There is also a variety of savoury food used in special occasions. One of them, Adas Polo is amazing, since it is considered to be one easiest Persian foods but with a bit of technique, turns into a very formal food.

It's also used on other occasions, like a more daily used food, but is are mostly known for those occasions. This version, with green lentils and rice is so popular, almost every family has it at least twice a month, mainly for lunch, especially because it's one of kids' favourite foods. Though if you're invited for the first time to an Iranian family's house as a guest, I doubt that they would cook Adas Polo for you unless you have asked for it.

The origin of Adas Polo is not clear, yet it became more popular after Safavi dynasty started extending religious ceremonies. In at least one of these ceremonies – Sham E Ghariban, the night that one of the prophets passed – this dish is the only food that is served. This is probably one of the reasons it was popular in other religious ceremonies too.

Adas Polo is fast to cook, especially if it's served with minced meat, and should always be cooked with green lentils.

Another reason for the popularity of this dish is that growing all sorts of lentil is increasingly popular among Iranian farmers. Lentils are reasonably priced compared to other grains. They are also fast to cook, which Iranians believe makes them easy to digest.

Serves 4

Cooking time: 1 hour

- 3 cups rice, washed and soaked with two tbsp of salt for two hours
- 300 grams minced meat (chicken, beef or lamb)
- 1 tbsp turmeric
- 3 tbsp salt
- 1 tsp black pepper
- 1.5 cups green lentils
- 2 tbsp vegetable oil
- 1 piece of flatbread or 1 potato, thinly sliced
- 150 grams butter
- 1 cup golden raisins, washed
- 150 grams dates
- Barberries (optional)
- 1 tsp saffron (brewed with ice or two tablespoons boiling water)
- 3 tbsp caramelised brown onion
- 1 tbsp ground cinnamon

Method

Heat vegetable oil on a low heat in a medium pan and add mince, turmeric, a third of a tablespoon of salt and pepper. Stir well. Add half a cup of boiling water, pop the lid on and cook for 30 minutes.

Wash lentils and cover with water and the rest of the salt in a pot on medium heat. Let the lentils cook for about 20 minutes, or until the lentils are soft enough to eat.

Fill 1/3 of another medium size pot with boiling water and place over a high heat. Once the water is boiling, rinse and add the rice, occasionally giving a gentle stir. Once the rice is soft on the outside and still hard inside it's time to drain the rice.

The minced meat will be cooked by now if the extra water is vaporised. Take off the heat

Take the lentils off the heat and drain separately.

Add two tablespoons oil to a medium size pan and leave flatbread or potatoes on the bottom. Using a spatula, layer one full spatula of rice and one full spatula of cooked lentils in turns until all rice and lentils are in the pot.

Push into the shape of a mountain peak and add few holes in the mound to vaporise the extra water. Drizzle with 50 grams of melted butter.

Wrap the lid with a clean tea towel and put the lid back on top of the top. Cook on a very low heat for 45 minutes.

While the rice is cooking, fry the raisins in 50 grams of butter in a small saucepan, stirring, for 15 seconds. Do the same in another small saucepan with the dates. (If you don't like the sweet taste, you can skip this step, but I strongly recommend it.) If you want to include barberries in your garnish, follow the same process again.

When the rice is ready, gently mix two tablespoons of rice with the brewed saffron.

To serve, add rice to a medium, flat serving plate in a round shape. Top with minced meat, then the fried raisins, dates and barberries, if using, and on the very top, add saffron rice, caramelised onions and cinnamon.

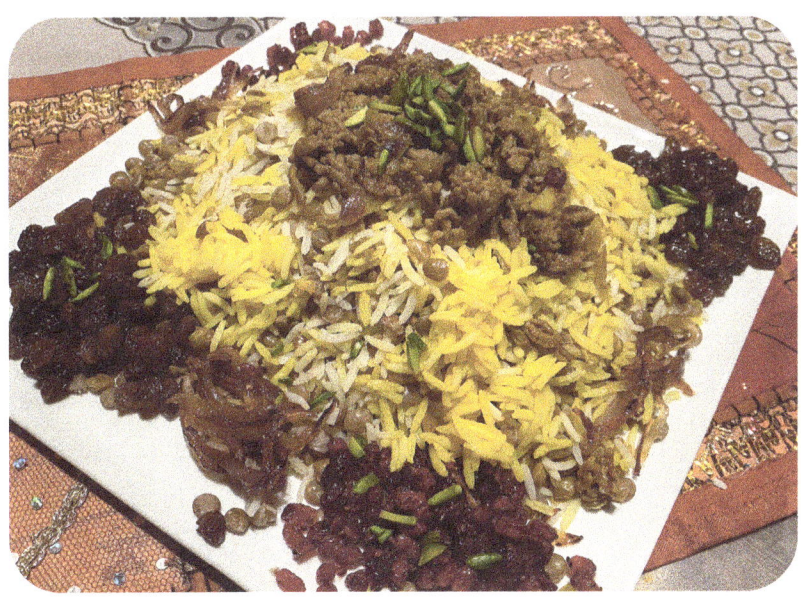

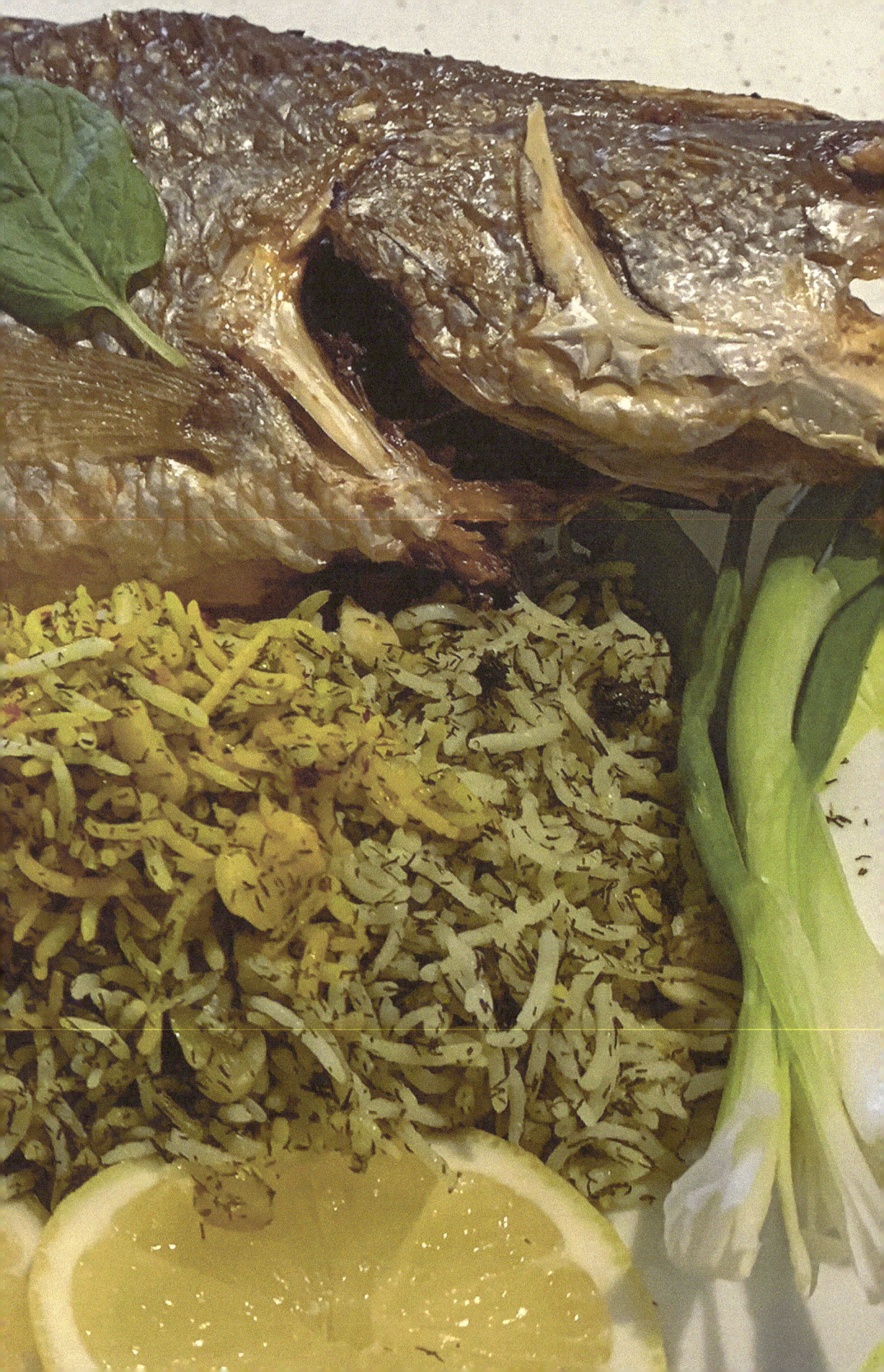

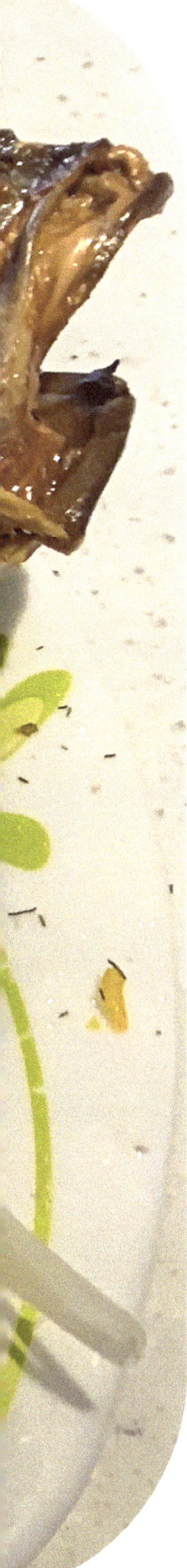

Sabzi Polo Mahi
(cooked rice with herbs and fried fish)

In Farsi, cooked rice which is soaked, half cooked, drained and cooked again is called Polo. Rice cooked in a rice cooker is called Kateh. Uncooked rice is called. Berenj. Having all these different names shows the importance of rice in Iranian life – rice and tea are the two products in the highest demand in Iran.

Sabzi Polo Mahi is the most famous Persian food, because this food is a reminder of a very famous national ceremony, Nowruz. Nowruz is the Iranian new year celebration which coincides with the first day of spring. It is a celebration to welcome spring and start of a new year, like celebrating the awakening of nature from winter's sleep. In the western calendar, the time for this event is sometime in February or March.

Nowruz has been the biggest Iranian ceremony for thousands of years, since the beginning of civilisation. It also celebrated by several other countries, including by Afghan people and people who live in Azabaijan, since these countries were all one country and all part of the Persian Empire. The celebration was always there, but some traditions, like eating Sabzi polo Mahi was latter added to the culture of celebrating. In ancient times only those with access to bodies of water would be able to harvest fish. This meant that people in the rest of the country had Sabzi Polo with another dish, probably Koko Sabzi (herb omelette). For us, these food are far more than just a celebration of new year, they are the identity of our nation.

Apart from the food, there is lots of excitement and other interesting traditions in Persian household during Nowruz.

The celebration actually starts almost twenty days before the big day, when everyone (and I really mean everyone) starts spring cleaning. The ancient Persians believed that cleaning their homes from top to bottom and getting rid of any trace of dust from the old year would get rid of any problems or bad luck they probably had during the last year. By coming into the new year in their clean house, they believed the best luck in life and destiny would happen to them.

Some people, who can afford it, not only do their spring cleaning but replace everything in their house, like furniture, with new things. So shopping is a big part of this ceremony. If you walk in streets few weeks before Nowruz you can feel a significant change in streets. Along every footpath, you will see temporary shops selling things and calling or singing to customers to attract their attention. Although this act is against local laws at other times of the year, things are different in this time of the year.

A few days before new year's eve, there is a very famous event in the early evening of the last Tuesday of the year. This is a kind of fireworks called Chahr Shanbeh Suri It's called Chahr Shanbeh (Wednesday), because Suri means red in Kurdish, as the fire which is very important part of this celebration is red. This is because before Islam become the country's formal religion, Iranian used to be Zartostian. For Zartostian, fire and its flame is something holy. They believe the flame of fire cleans everything, warms their homes, cooks their foods, and gives light to its surroundings. On the night of Chahr Shanbeh Suri, people make small flames with little pieces of firewood in streets, and jump over that fire to protect themselves with the power of that flame in coming year.

Then, the night before Nowruz is the night usually people gather with their immediate relatives and have dinner together which is always Sabzi Polo Mahi. No matter in which state or what house you drop into that night, every family all over the country will be serving their family this same dish.

The herbs in this dish represent the green of spring and trees starting new life. The rice is representing being blessed with food in coming year and the fish is representing life in new the year.

Now, I will tell you the story why we eat this food. Solomon the prophet had a magic ring, and he could make all demons and angels obey him with this ring. One day, a giant ogre found the prophet's ring by chance, and mesmerised everyone with the power of the ring to make them believe he was Solomon, the king and prophet. When people believed him, the ogre kicked the real Solomon out of town and threw the ring into the sea so no one could find out was not the real Solomon. The real Solomon couldn't convince people he is the real one, so he started fishing to find the ring, opening each fish to find the ring. He did that for many many years until he found the ring. Solomon came back to his kingdom on the last day of the Nowruz ceremony, which was the thirteenth day of the first month of spring. With that ring, Solomon could prove the reality and took back his kingdom. Since the fish was the cause for revealing the reality it became a tradition for people to believe eating fish will reveal reality to them.

In these old days, Iranian had a special place for greens. They believed they must eat something green the night before the start of the new year because green is representing new life and blessing. They also believed that by eating something green, their agriculture industry for next year would be blessed and their products will grow green and good.

Those who couldn't afford fish used to eat their herbs and rice with a KoKo (a sound that comes from poultry as it had eggs in it) Sabzi (herbs).

So, here we have the recipes for these three dishes but since they are usually eaten together, they are kind of like one dish.

Sabzi Polo (herbs and rice)

Serves 4

Prep time: 20 minutes

Cooking time: 45

- 2 cups long grain basmati rice, washed and soaked with two tbsp of salt for at two hours
- 1/4 cup fresh dill, washed and chopped
- 1/4 cup fresh chives, washed and chopped

- 1/4 cup fresh parsley, washed and chopped
- 1/4 cups fresh coriander, washed and chopped
- 2 tbsp fresh garlic, chopped
- 2 tbsp vegetable oil
- 2 tbsp butter
- 2 tbsp salt

Method

Fill 1/3 of medium pot with water and bring to the boil. When the water is boiling, add soaked rice. The rice is half cooked when if you take one grain of rice between two fingers it looks cooked from outside but when you break it, it looks still raw from the inside. Drain the rice.

Mix all chopped herbs and garlic in a separate bowl.

In another pot, pour two tablespoons of vegetable oil, add one layer of drained rice and one layer of the mixed herbs. Continue layering until all rice and herbs are in the pot. Make the mixture look like a mountain peak and make one big hole in the middle of the peak. Melt the butter and pour on top. Wrap with a clean tea towel and the lid, and put the pot back on a low heat for 45 minutes (make sure tea towel is safely covering the lid, so when you put pot on the heat, the tea towel is not in any contact with the heat).

Hashoo (stuffed and baked fish)

For this dish, the fish (any you desire) is washed, cleaned and marinated and then simply deep fried. You probably know how to deep fry a fish, so here I take the opportunity to introduce you to special fish frying recipe – Hashoo. This is common in southern Iran, which you can eat either with plain rice or with Sabzi Polo Mahi. Hashoo could be considered a sauce for fish. In local language, hashoo means stuffing – usually used with the use special kind of fish that local fishermen from southern cities catch from sea, close to the Persian Gulf – but it goes well with any other kind of fish too. Fish with firmer textures, like snapper, are best for this recipe.

Serves 4 (though this depends on the size of your chosen fish)

- Prep time: 20 minutes
- Cooking time: 40 minutes

- 1 medium firm fish, washed
- 2 bunches fresh coriander, washed and finely chopped
- 1/2 bunch fresh fenugreek, washed and finely chopped or 1 tbsp dried fenugreek
- 1 large onion, finely chopped and caramelised
- 8 cloves garlic, finely chopped
- 1 tbsp turmeric
- 1/4 tsp red chilli powder
- 250 grams tamarind purée
- Salt, to taste
- 2 tbsp olive oil, vegetable oil or melted butter

Method

Combine chopped herbs, onion, garlic, spices, tamarind purée and salt.

Cut fish from its belly to top to make one flat piece.

Rub melted butter on inside surface of fish.

Put the mixture of herbs, spices and tamarind purée over all inside surface of fish.

Turn the oven to 180 degrees and bake the fish with skin side down for 30 minutes. For grilling do the same, and leave fish on grill from skin side.

Serve with either plain rice or with Sabzi Polo.

Koko Sabzi (herb omelette)

98 per cent of the time we are cooking Sabzi Polo Mahi, it comes with Koko Sabzi. As I said earlier, in the old days only people living close to the water had access to fresh fish, so on the new year's night this was sitting on the table next to Sabzi Polo.

But we Iranians don't know how deeply we have fallen in love with this dish. It's mostly cooked by busy mums, board students, herb and vegetarian food lovers and for kids' lunches or sometimes, for breakfast. Or for busy days when you're wanting something fast yet delicious.

Usually, any fajita cooked with egg is called Koko. There is a big variety of Koko in Persian cuisine but among them Koko Sabzi and Koko seib zamin (potato omelette) are the favourites. It is also very common to eat these without rice, with bread as a sandwich. They will go with any kind of side, but fresh lettuce leaves or sliced fresh tomato are best.

I strongly suggest using only fresh herbs, but if you find a pack of frozen Koko sabzi herbs in a Persian shop this would work okay too.

Serves 6

Cooking time: 50 minutes (20 minutes for each side)

- 2 bunches of fresh parsley, washed and finely chopped
- 1 bunch fresh chives, washed and finely chopped
- 1 bunch fresh coriander, washed and finely chopped
- 6 eggs
- 1 1/2 tsp salt
- 1 tsp ground black pepper
- 1 tbsp flour
- 1/3 tsp turmeric
- 2 tbsp walnuts, crushed
- 1/2 cup vegetable oil
- 2 tbsp barberries, washed
- 4–5 lettuce leaves, chopped

Method

In a large bowl mix all chopped herbs. Break the eggs into this mix and add salt, pepper, turmeric, flour and walnuts. Whisk well.

Heat vegetable oil in a Teflon pan with a lid (do not use an aluminium pan) a on medium heat. To check if the oil is hot enough, hold a wooden spoon in the oil. If the oil starts sizzling, it's hot enough.

Gently add half the mixture to the pan, making sure it is even on all sides and wait for 7 to 9 minutes. Then, add barberries evenly to the surface (but not close to edges) and gently add the rest of the mixture to the pan to cover barberries.

Put the lid on and leave for at least 20 minutes on a low to medium heat.

Gently transfer to a bigger pan and flip it upside down to cook the other side. on the same heat for another 20 minutes. (If flipping it over is hard for you, once you've added the second layer to cover the barberries, you can cook in the oven at 175 degrees for 15 to 20 minutes.)

Take off the heat or out of the oven. Wait for five minutes before cutting into slices like you would usually cut a cake.

If eating with bread, wrap slices in flatbread with desired sides. If eating with rice, each slice could simply be eaten with desired amount of rice

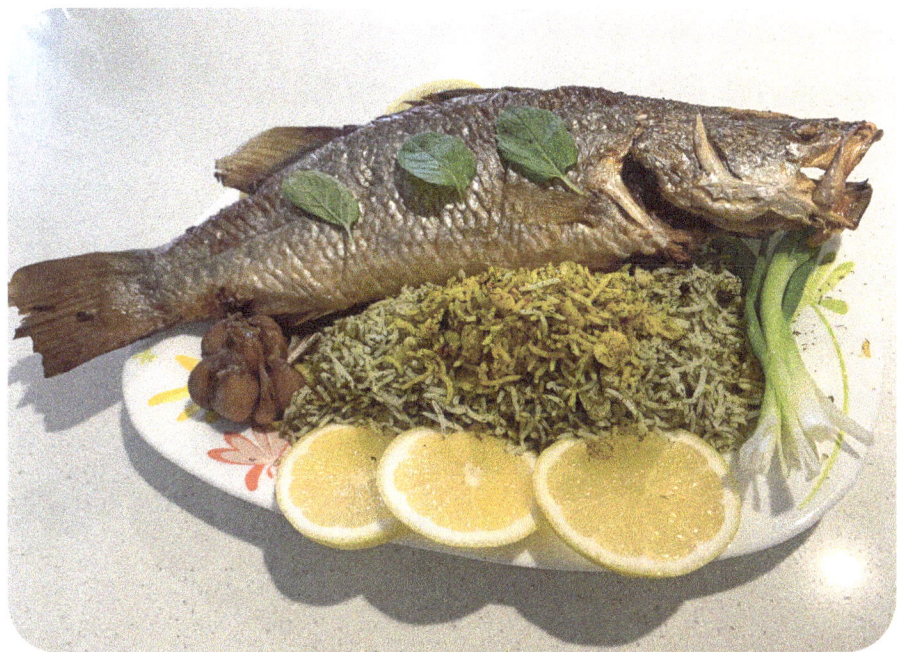

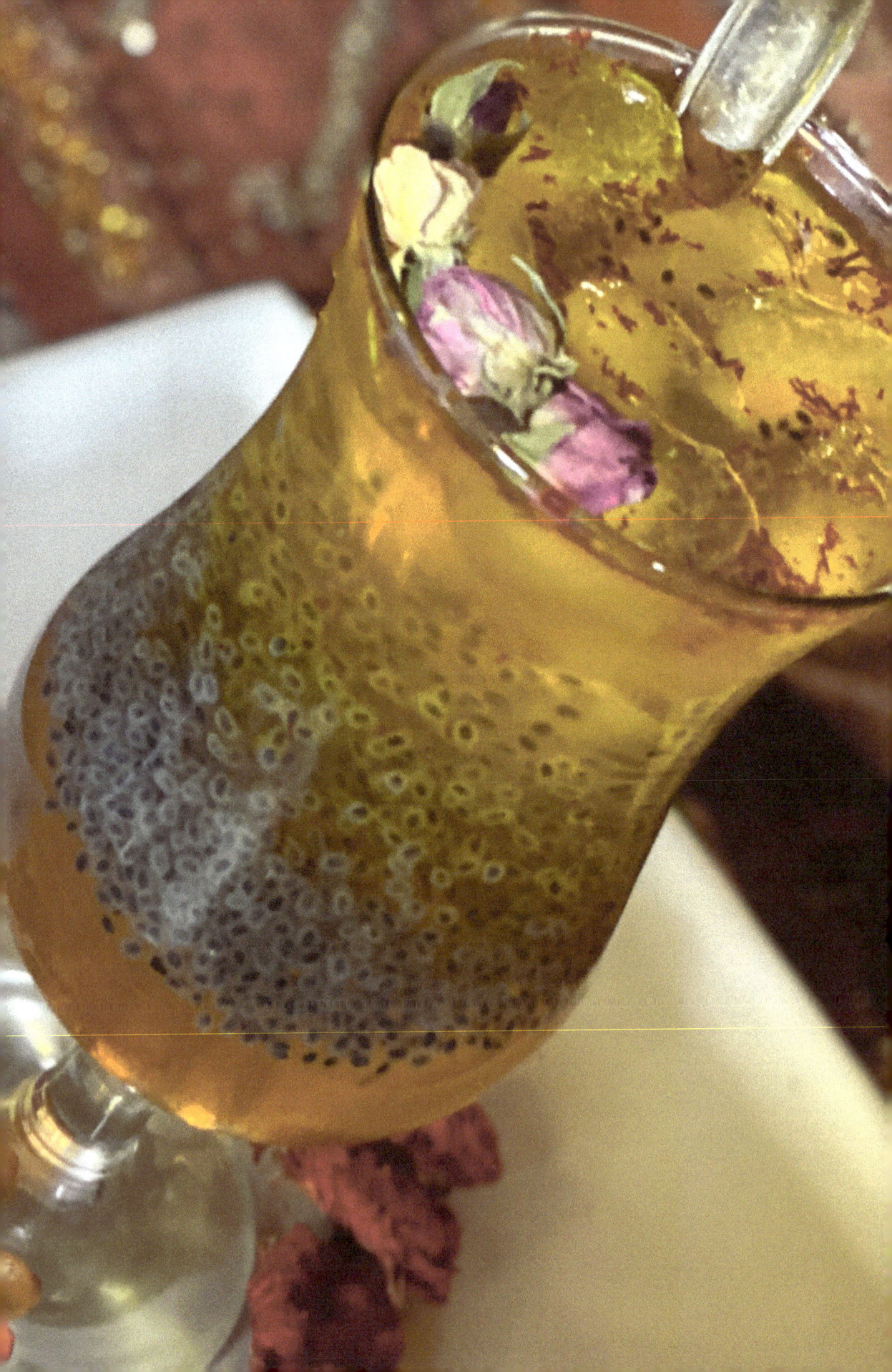

Saffron drink with basil seed and rose water

The next food which has ceremonial background is a drink: a very pleasant, unusual drink with lots of herbal benefits.

As I said earlier, there are number of religious ceremonies in the Iranian calendar which are very important and are respectably taken very serious by Iranians. Some of them are public holidays, and even most main streets are closed, with only people who are responsible for holding these ceremonies are allowed to pass those streets.

People who had made deals with God during the year make wishes, and if their wishes come true., they serve special kinds of food in the streets. If these ceremonies coincide with hot summer days, they serve a special kind of drink which you mostly only see being served during that time of year. If the ceremonies coincide with the cold season, they serve either with tea or hot chocolate.

As this drink has saffron in it, which is very common in Iran, it is believed this drink will come with lots of herbal benefits. You might know that Iran is the origin of saffron and is the biggest exporter of this amazing spice. The reason saffron is so expensive is that it can be only grown in soil with specific climate specifications, there is a very hard process of growing and cultivation and only few days in whole year in which it can be picked.

To work out if saffron is real or fake, there are number of tests you can go through. Real saffron has scent of sweetness: put one of the saffron threads in your mouth, and if in the beginning it tastes sweet but at the end has a strong bitter taste, that means that the saffron is real. Another test is to smell it: real saffron smells like honey. To store saffron at home, keep it a dark, cool place – usually the fridge is a good choice!

Serves 4

Prep time: 30 minutes

- 4 glasses cold water
- Juice of 1 fresh lemon
- 3 tbsp basil seeds
- 1/3 tsp saffron powder brewed with ice (just add ice cubes to powdered saffron and leave at least for 15 minutes)
- Sugar (amount will depend on how sweet you like the drink)
- 3 tbsp rose water

Method

Cover basil seeds with water in a big bowl and change the water few times to wash away any dust away.

Add sugar to the four cups of cold water and mix well until sugar is dissolved. Add brewed saffron and washed basil seeds.

Add lemon juice and mix well.

Add rose water and mix well. Serve while it's cold.

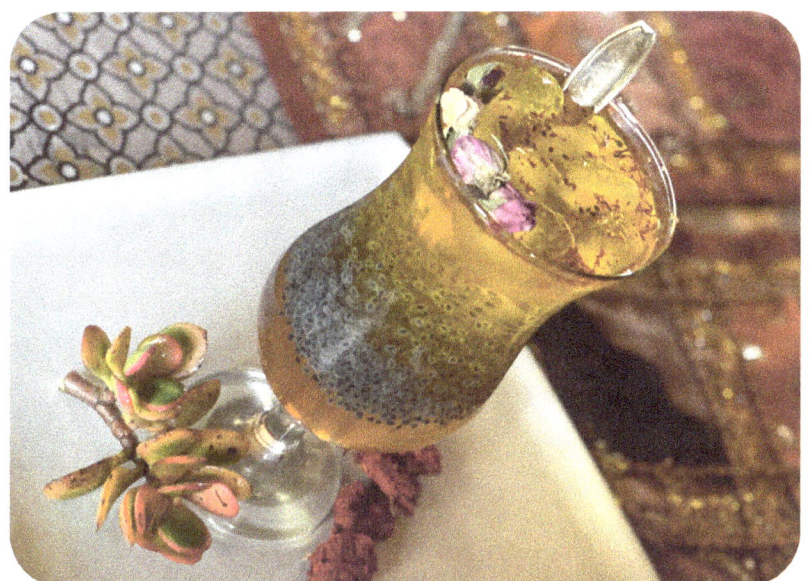

Food kids love

Like every other nation, Iranians are also concerned about kids not eating well. But it used to be exactly the opposite in the old days.

Since large numbers of people in the community were struggling to provide food for their families, kids used to be good at eating everything. In fact they used to eat anything, if it was available.

These days, Iranian kids are a little more fussy. But there are some cuisines among Iranian food that kids will never say no to.

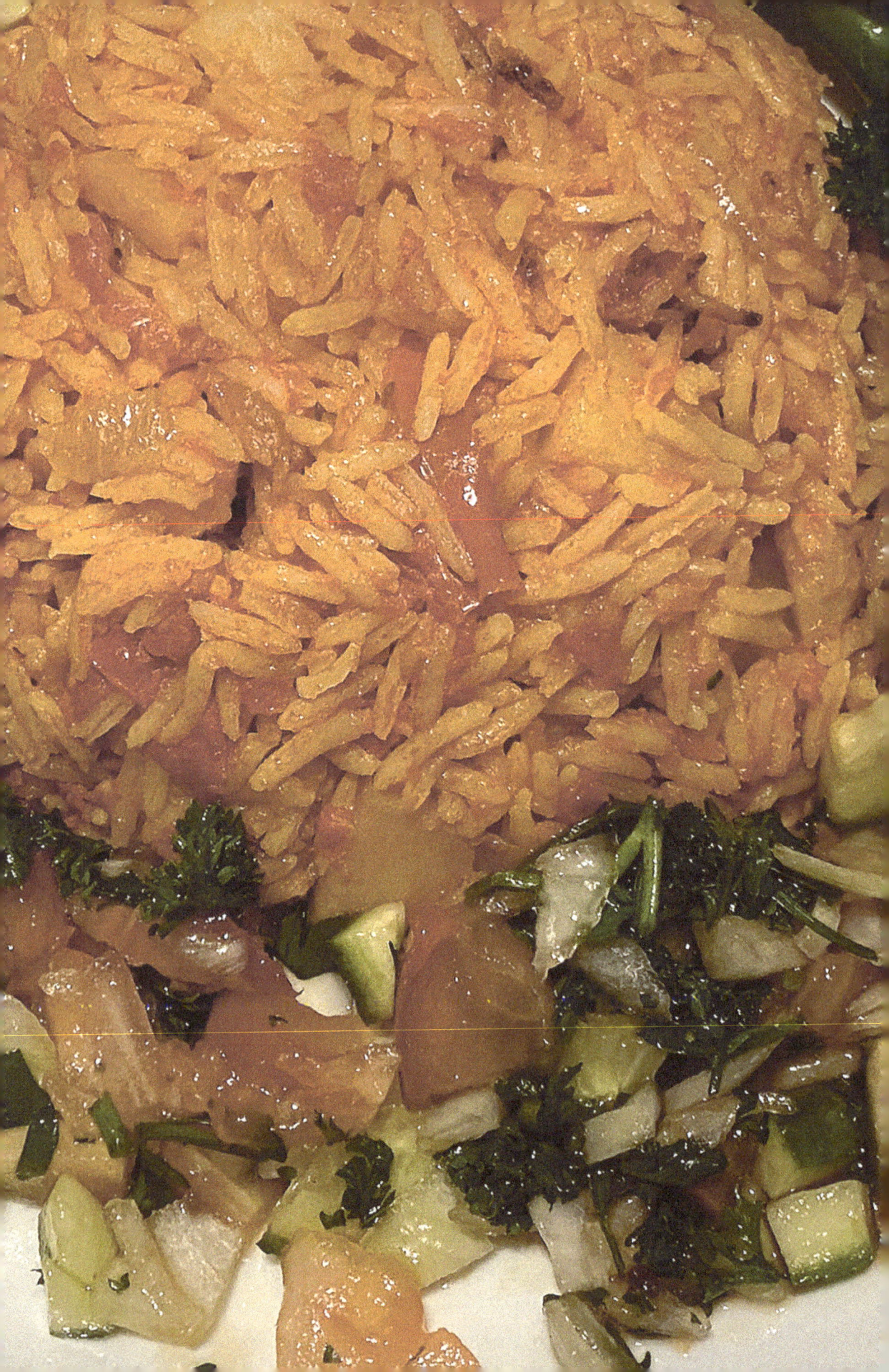

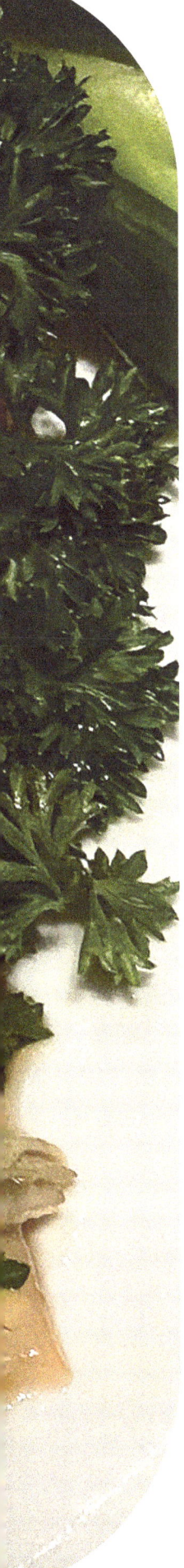

Istanbuli polo

One of Iran's ambassadors in Turkey, Mooshir O Dooleh, was ambassador in Istanbul for a long time during the Qajar dynasty. After a long time, the King of Iran asked him to return to Iran, as he wanted to grant him a higher position as a minister.

When he came back to country, Mooshir O Dooleh invited the King and his entourage for lunch in his home to celebrate his new position. Every time there was such an invitation – either for lunch or dinner – the King should be the first one at the table. So, the King came to the table to be served, where he saw a new dish among all the Persian cuisine. He found this dish – Istanbuli (from Istanbul) polo (rice) – very delicious.

The King loved Istanbuli polo so much that he ordered the court chef to learn and cook it in court. Soon, everyone in the court loved it so much and asked their home chefs to cook it for them too.

I've hardly met any kids who don't love Istanbuli polo. If in Iran, parents are faced with their kid's bad eating habits, they know that they will never say no to Istanbuli polo. Its easy preparation and cooking is also another reason that this food is so popular among Iranians of all ages.

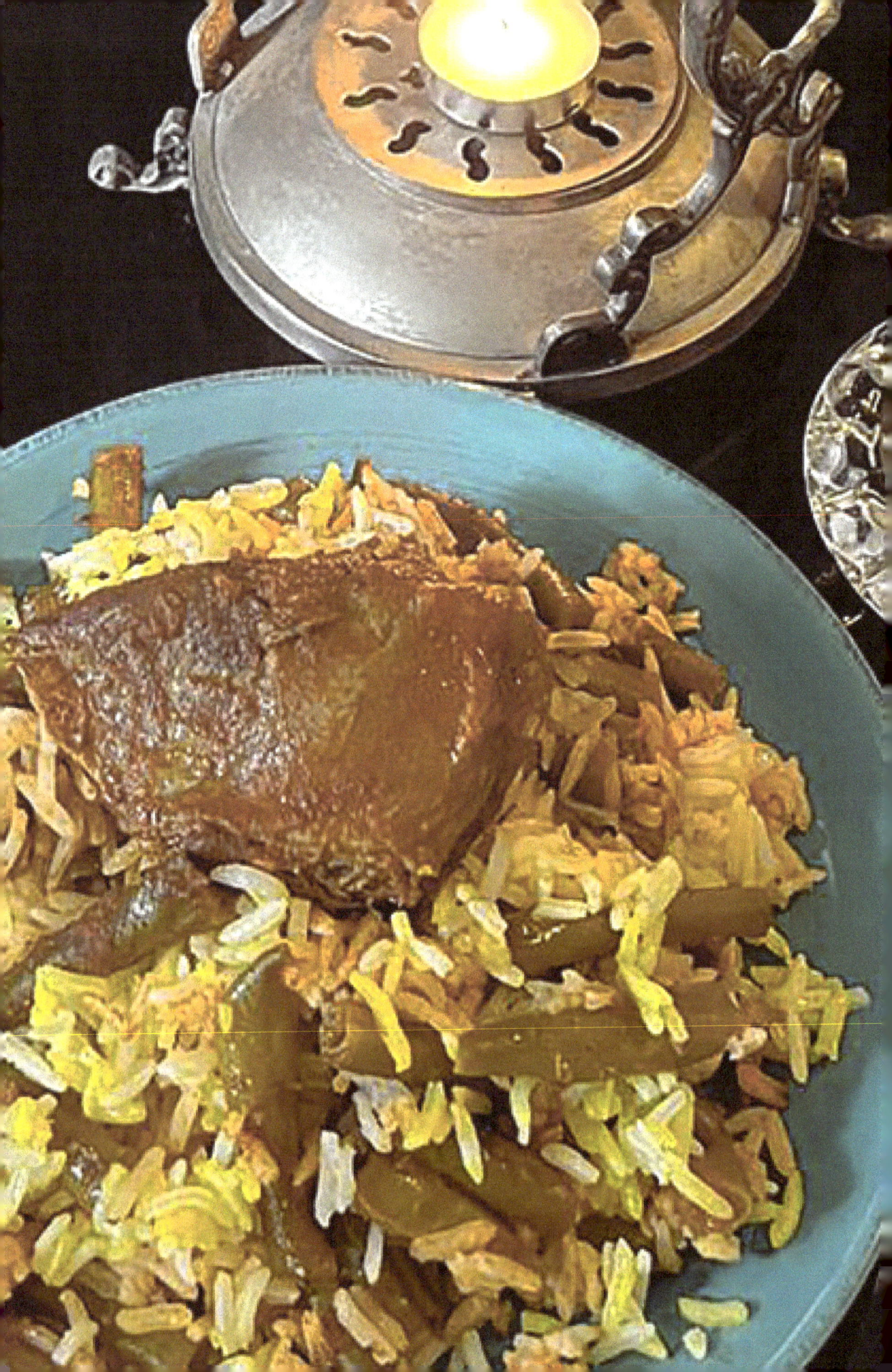

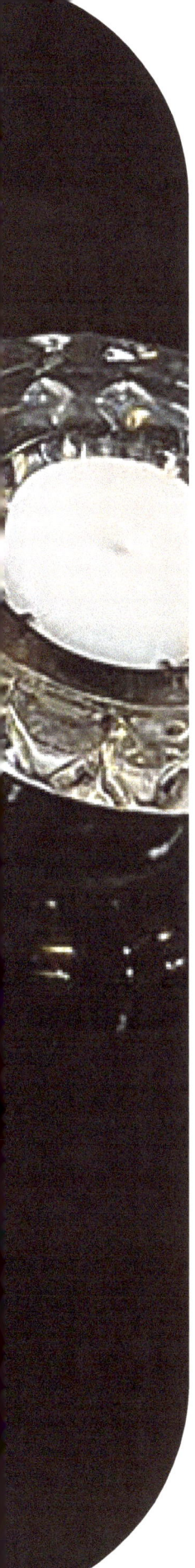

Loobiya Polo

Another dish I've personally never found a kid to say no to is loobiya polo. If you ask any Iranian about their childhood memories, you will definitely hear about loobiya polo. The amazing thing about this dish is that you continue to love it just the same even when you have grown up. It is not usually considered a restaurant dish but since it's so popular among kids there is a chance that some restaurants serve it too.

Like Istanbuli polo, loobiya polo is another souvenir dish from Iran's neighbour, Turkey. States in the north west of Iran share borders with Russia and Turkey. This means more travellers from these countries, who bring their culture and traditions as souvenirs.

When people from Turkey travelled to Iran both two countries exchanged a lot of traditions, including recipes, and loobiya polo was one of them.

Loobiya polo can be a bit of a risky rice dish. As I mentioned earlier, it's very important for Iranians that their rice lays nicely on the serving plate. Each grain of cooked rice, which they call polo, must be separated from other grain and not be gluey. Since there is sauce in mixture of green beans and meat, you must be aware of the right time to drain the rice, otherwise it will turn gluey.

Loobiya polo can cooked with diced or minced beef, lamb or chicken. For a vegetarian option, you can completely skip the meat or cook with soya.

If you have picky kids at home, I can guarantee they are going to love it.

Serves 4

Prep and cooking time: 1 hour 45 minutes

- 2 cups long grain basmati rice
- 1 medium onion, chopped
- 300 grams diced or minced beef, or lamb or chicken
- 200 grams green beans, washed and cut into 1 inch-pieces
- 3 tbsp tomato paste
- 1/2 tsp powdered saffron, brewed with either ice or boiling water (not both)
- 1/2 piece of Lebanese flatbread or one potato, sliced
- 1 tsp turmeric
- 1 tsp black pepper
- 1/2 tsp cinnamon
- Salt to taste
- Vegetable oil
- Water

Method

Soak rice with water and salt two hours in advance.

Fry onion in a medium size pan. When colour started to change, add diced or minced meat, turmeric, salt, pepper and tomato paste. Stir and leave for a few minutes

Add water to covers the mixture and leave on medium heat.

In another pan, fry the cut green beans in two tablespoons of oil, stirring occasionally for about 10 minutes. Add green beans to the other pan leave it until both the meat and beans are cooked well.

When more than half of all the liquid is vaporised, remove from the heat. The sauce should be thick and tender.

Fill a medium size pot with one third of water and bring to the boil. When the water is boiling, add the soaked rice. When rice looks on third cooked (it should still look kind of but not too raw – like each grain is half soft on the outside but still hard inside), drain the rice in cold water.

In another medium size pan, pour two tablespoons of oil. Lay one layer of either flatbread pieces or thin slices of potato pieces in the bottom of the pot.

Over the flatbread or potatoes, add one or two layers of drained rice and one layer of cooked beans and meat. Continue layering same until all mixtures are in the pot.

Make rice look like a mountain peak in the pot by bring it to the centre from sides using a wooden spoon.

Using the handle of a wooden spoon, make one big hole in the centre of the rice to steam the rice while it's cooking.

Scatter cinnamon on top of the rice.

Wrap the lid with a clean tea towel to absorb extra vaporised water from rice (that helps the rice to hold its shape from going gluey).

Leave on a low heat for at least 45 minutes.

When you are ready to serve and are transferring rice from the pot to serving plate, melt one tablespoon of butter, ghee or vegetable oil and drizzle over the rice.

When all of the cooked green beans and rice are in the plate, gently take out the crispy flatbread or potatoes, and serve them on another plate. This crispy layer is called Tah (bottom) Dig (pot): this is the part of food that family members always fight over and the favourite part of every Persian rice dish. It actually has its own very interesting story, which we will read in further chapters.

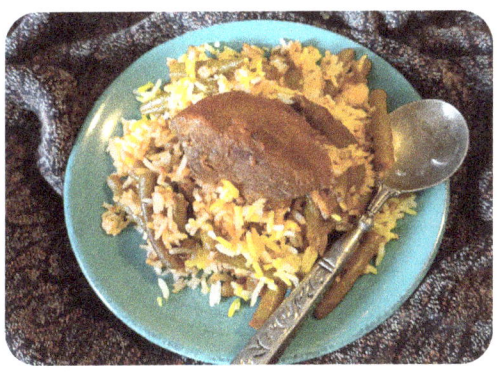

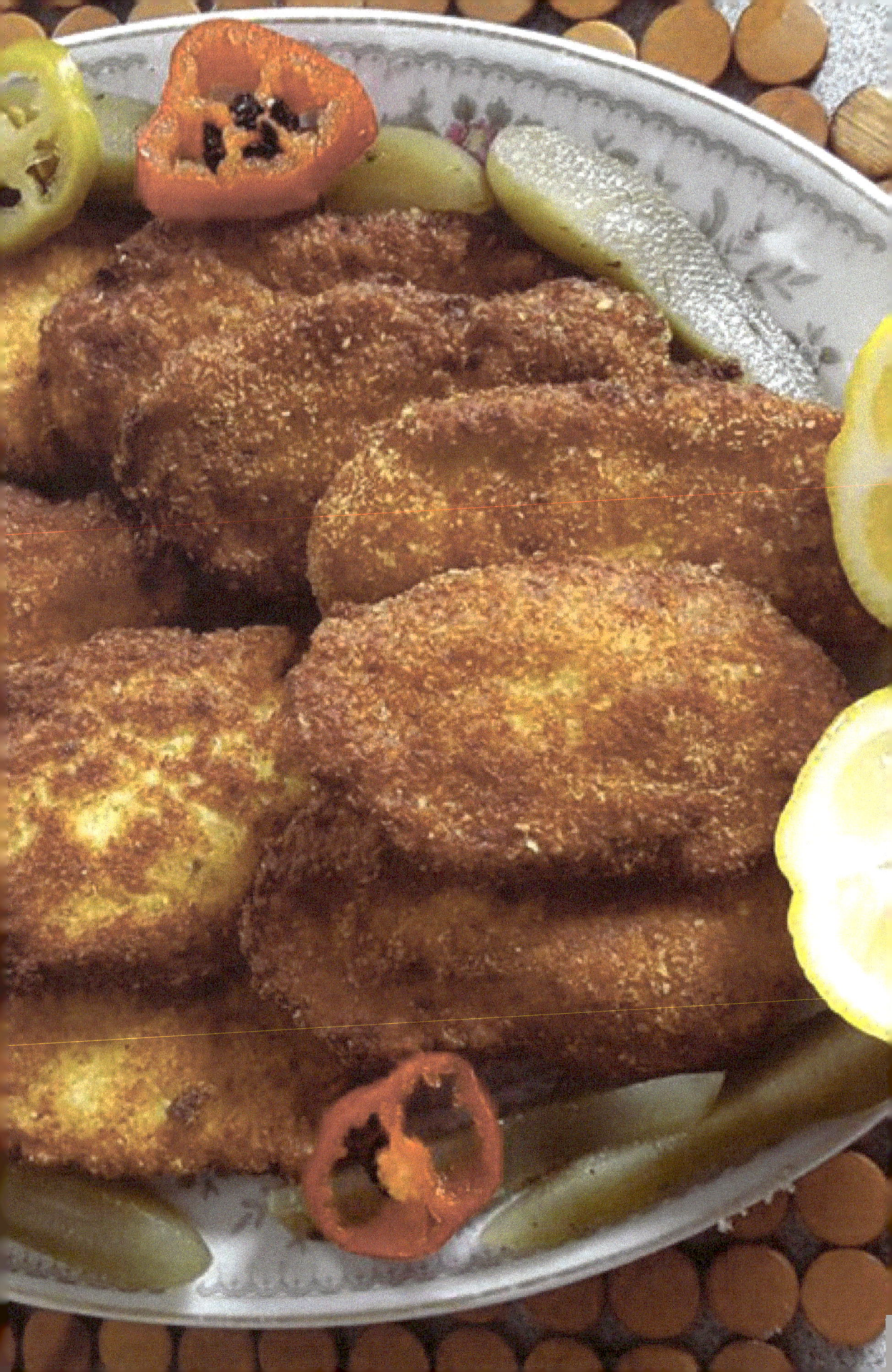

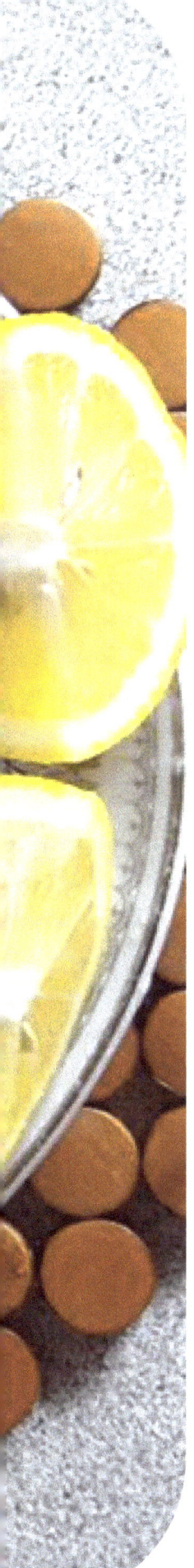

Kotlet
(Persian patties)

Once you have tried Kotlet, you would believe it's not only kids favourite Persian food, but the whole world's favourite. For a lot of us it's not only a food, but a time machine to flash back to your childhood.

I remember when I was kid, every time we went camping with family and friends we kids used to play with stones and mud near rivers. I used to mix the muds with water to pretending I'm making Kotlet dough and cooking it for my mates playing with me. A lot of the time when we were playing, we would pretend to cook this dish – probably because the acts of pretending to cook this food could feel more real compared to other imaginary foods.

As Middle Eastern girls, especially in my generation, we knew that cooking was probably the first and most important thing we needed to learn as women. I don't know whether it's a good or bad sign but the younger generations have been through significant changes about these ideas. Now, like every other country, women in the Middle East are more involved with society's affairs but still you can find girls who are following both patterns.

Kotlet is among the Persian foods served with flatbread and sides. It's also considered a street food, but for some reason people prefer to homemade versions, maybe because of the mixture needing to be made by hand, and they trust homemade ones more.

With only slight differences in ingredients (like more spices, and less meat) and shape of cooking it would be called Shami which originated in India. For Kotlet, meat is considered the hero ingredient.

The other fun thing about Kotlet is since they are pieces of dough fried in oil, almost all Iranian kids have experienced asking their mums to make a little for them, and that's how mums capture their kids heart every time they cook Kotlet.

Kotlet is also the number one choice for picnics and camping, as people usually prepare it in advance at home. It's also easy to carry as it doesn't need to be taken in pots and just as delicious cold, so or doesn't necessarily need to be warmed up like other Persian foods. In this case, it's always prepared the night before – for such foods, Iranians say the food becomes Bayat (stale) – but for some food like Kotlet or Shami some believe it's even more tasty when it's stale. For the same reasons, it's also very popular for informal parties and birthday parties.

Kotlet is usually served as a wrap with salty cucumber pickle and tomato slices, and sometimes fresh herbs or lettuce leaves. Of course, these sides were Kotlet's mates long before people were introduced to tomato sauce!

Serves 4

Prep and cooking time: 1 hour

- 250 grams minced beef or chicken
- 2 large potatoes
- 1 medium onion
- 1 tsp turmeric
- 1 tsp black pepper
- 1 tsp of salt
- 1 egg
- 2 cloves garlic, minced
- Vegetable oil, for frying

Method

Boil one potato and grate it into a large bowl. In another bowl, grate the other peeled raw potato and throw away excess liquid. (There are two different ways of cooking Kotlet: one with boiled potatoes and one is with grated raw potatoes, but in my experience the best result comes preparing one each way.)

Mix boiled and raw potatoes together.

Grate the onion and throw away excess liquid. Add to the potatoes.

Add mince, turmeric, salt, pepper, garlic and egg (if you like, you can add some more spices like minced ginger or cumin powder, depending on your taste and your creativity. Even some dried herbs could be good but they are not in the original recipe.)

Mix well until it has a consistent texture. If you find the mixture a bit runny or too wet add one tablespoon of breadcrumbs and mix well again.

Leave the dough to rest for at least one hour.

Heat enough oil to fry the Kotlet (without covering whole the Kotlet) in a large pan over a medium heat.

Using a bowl of cold water next to you, wet your hands and take about two tablespoons of dough in your hand. Pat it into a flat patty (not too thick or thin). Repeat until you have used up all the dough.

Check the oil to see if it's hot enough with bottom of wooden spoon (when it's hot enough, the spoon will start sizzling).

Wash your hands and place patties gently into the hot oil. Once the edges turn golden brown, flip them over to fry the other side. Gently add more oil if needed.

Place a dish with paper towel next to your work station to absorb the excess oil from the fried patties.

Garnish with thin slices of salty cucumber pickle, tomato and red onion slices. Serve with flatbread.

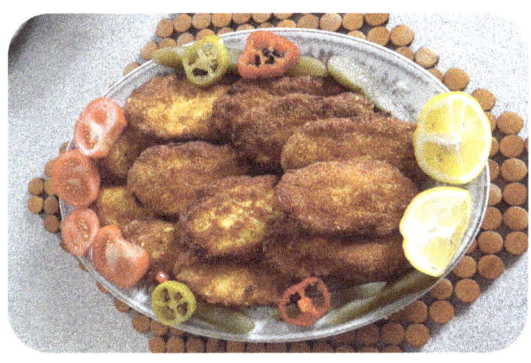

Food with medical benefits

In Iranian culture, foods are divided in two categories for their nature: food with hot nature and food with cold nature. People are divided into these two categories too.: People with white and fair skin are considered to be cold in nature and people with dark skin are considered to be hot in nature.

For example, people living in southern Iran, where there is strong sun and hot weather, have mostly dark skin, which comes from spending too much time in and getting burned by the hot sun. On the other hand, people from northern Iran, where there is lots of rain and less sun, have white skin so their nature must be cold.

Anyway, according to this division those with hot nature must eat more food with cold nature (like watermelon) and vice versa. Likewise, if you have been eating lots of food with cold nature, you should eat food which is with hot nature, like garlic, to bring balance to your body.

No one knows these food categories perfectly, but in some areas, especially older generations, people follow it religiously.

In Iran, there a large numbers of herbal medicine pharmacies all over the country. In the past, most of the people running these pharmacies just learned how, when and what to use from their ancestors but now to run such pharmacies you need to be accredited herbal medicine doctor or traditional medicine professional, having done a course at university.

It is believed the benefits of these herbal medicines can be experienced through some foods in Iranian cuisine, and I am going to point to a few of them here.

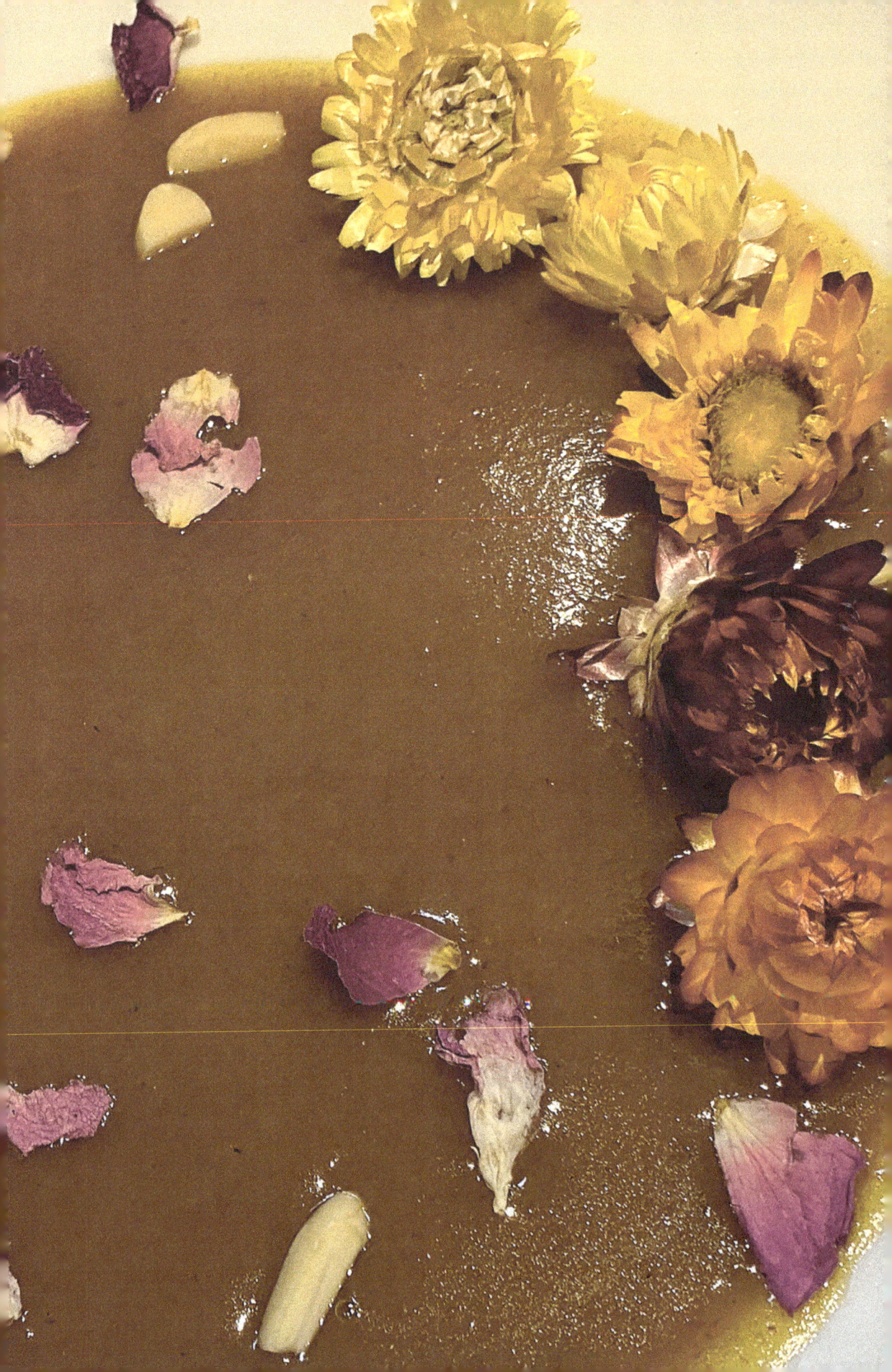

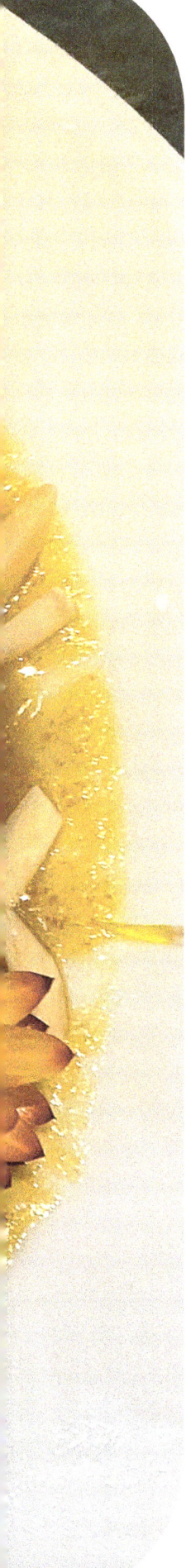

Kachi

No one really knows whether Kachi is a food, dessert or medicine. If it's a medicine, I guarantee you have never tasted a medicine as delicious as this one.

Kachi is well known among different states, with different reputation from state to state. In some states, it is considered a traditional food from a religious point of view, and is served in religious occasions.

In some states, it is believed that this is a food that should always be cooked and eat by women as Muslims have few women prophets. So, they follow special traditional steps while they're cooking, like reading some special words from their holy book or reciting some special poems to praise their women prophets. No men are allowed to be present at the time of cooking, to hear their voice, and the final product is never offered to men.

More commonly among almost all states, it's a special food given to women who have just given birth. When cooked for women after giving birth, some spices might be added too as they believe giving birth changes the nature of body to a cold nature, so a few hot nature spices must be added to

Kachi to return back your nature to hot nature. Women also lose a lot of blood when giving birth, and they need these hot nature spices to reproduce the lost blood in their body. Every person who comes to greet this new mum should eat a small plate of Kachi to share her happiness.

Kachi is also commonly prepared for the bride and groom the day after a marriage ceremony, as their first breakfast in their married life. In this instance, it has another requirement too. While the priest is reading the traditional marriage words, young women rub two pieces of hard sugar on top of the bride's head while her head is covered with a clean and white piece of fabric. It's believed these young girls are rubbing sweetness and happiness onto the bride head and that will make her marriage sweet. The powder that comes from the rubbing sugar must be use as the main ingredient in the Kachi prepared for the bride and groom, to add to the love between them.

Sometimes, the bride's family is responsible for providing the first breakfast for the couple. In this case, this breakfast is very heavy to show the bride's family's love and respect for the new couple. Kachi is the main dish in this breakfast along with other foods, like the best quality cheese, butter, heavy cream, honey, different kinds of jam and freshly baked bread.

Kachi is also recommended for people who have been in recovery from a surgery or from any physical difficulties. It's also believed to re-energise the body or good for women who have difficult periods.

Serves 6

Cooking time: 40 minutes

- 2 cups sugar
- 1 tsp saffron
- 1 cup wheat flour (this could be changed to rice flour to make Kachi gluten-free, but in this case, you might need to stir more as the colour of rice flour changes later when fried)
- 1/2 tsp ground cardamon
- 300 grams butter or ghee
- 1/5 cup vegetable oil
- 1/2 cup rose water
- 10 cups water

Method

To make syrup, add sugar to two glass of water and cook in a pot. When the syrup starts to thicken (though the syrup should not be very thick) add the saffron. Turn off the heat and set aside.

Start frying flour by itself in a medium pan on low to medium heat, gently stirring. Once the flour starts to darken, first add cardamon (in some states they add cinnamon and ginger powder too), then butter or ghee. Keep stirring and let colour go a bit darker. Add the oil, then water, continuing to stir finally add syrup.

Continue stirring until the mixture starts getting medium thick (but not very thick) like a soup. Add rose water, stir for a few more seconds and turn off the heat.

Kachi can be served hot or cold but is usually served cold garnished with slivered almonds and pistachios and dried rose petals.

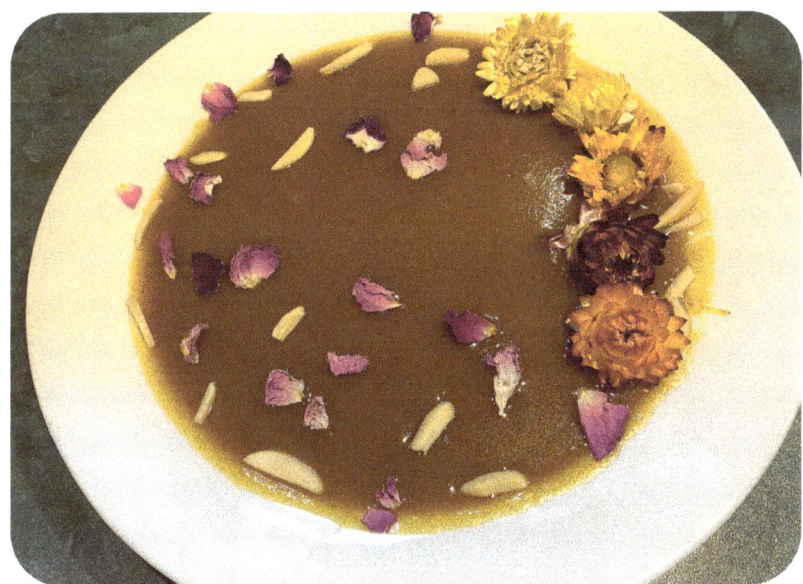

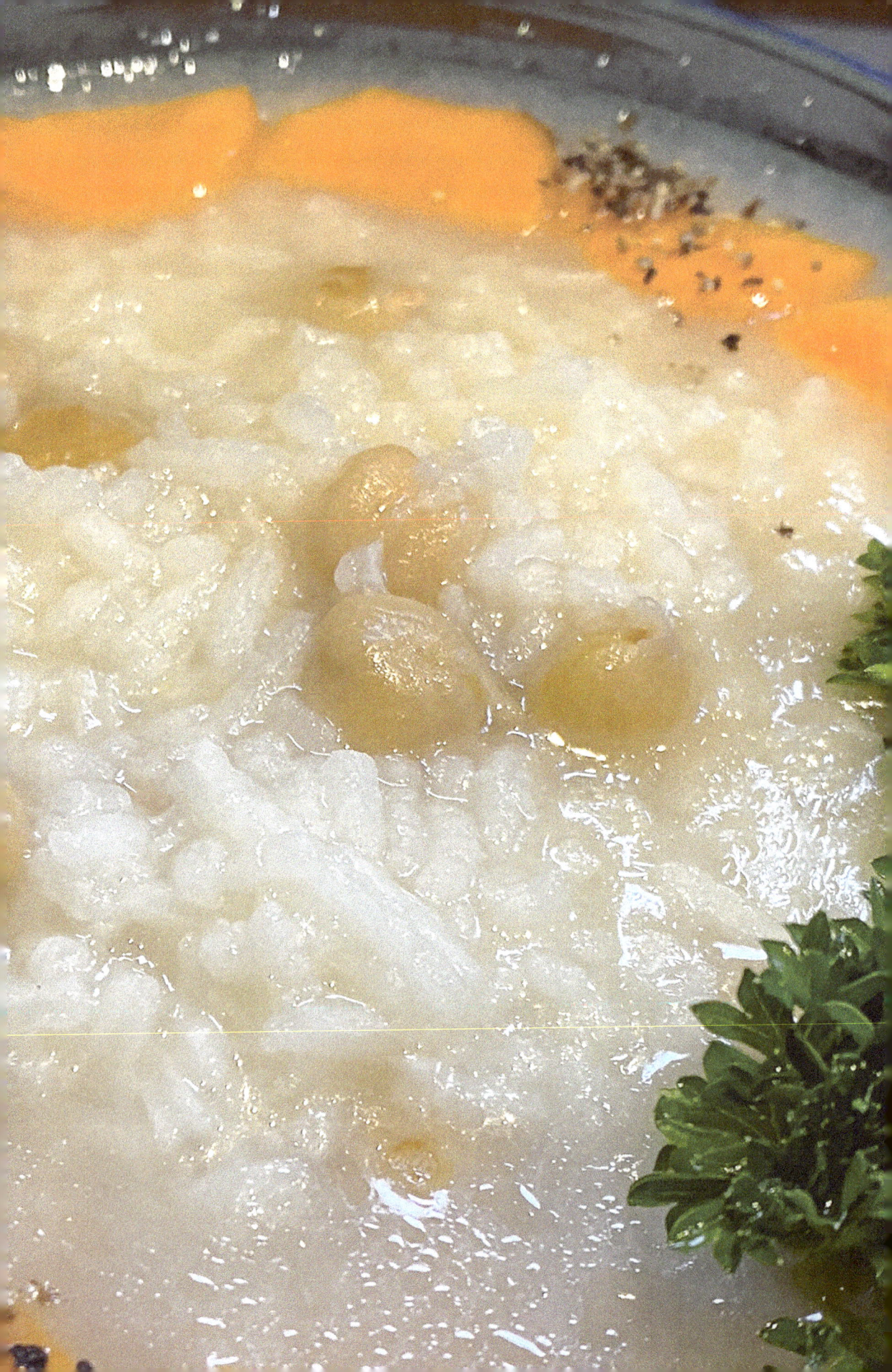

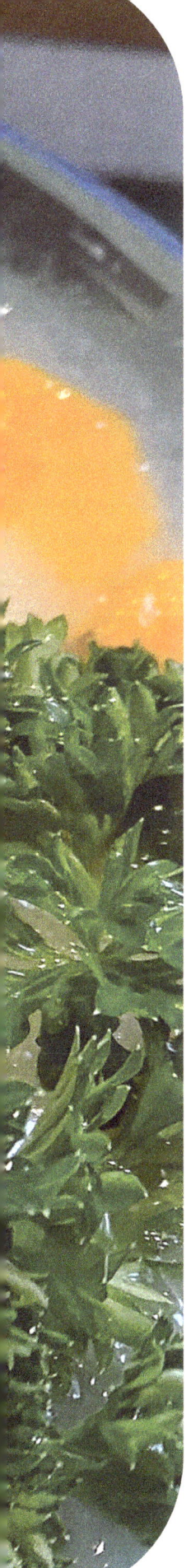

Chickpea soup

As western food arrived in Iranian homes, people started using less grains. Grains used to have a very special place in Iranian culture – not only from nutritional point of view but also for their medical benefits. No other grain or beans have been more the centre of attention than chickpeas.

Wild chickpea are small and black and could be find in remote mountainous areas but white chickpeas are more commonly used.

The origin of this soup is not clear but it used to be eaten very widely among different states, especially when someone was in recovery from hard health problems.

Given the division of foods into cold and hot categories, it is also believed that the root of all diseases and damage in the human immune system is because of cold body nature. In some special situation, your body might shift from one to the other –like if you have hot nature and you give a birth to a baby boy, your body might shift to being cold in nature and that sudden shift may affect your health. In cases like this, you must eat food with hot nature to bring balance to your body.

This chickpeas soup is considered to fall into the hot nature category. It's mostly only cooked if someone in the house is feeling unwell.

Serves 4

Cooking time: 3 to 4 hours

- 400 grams dried chickpeas, soaked for at least 4 hours
- 1 bone marrow, broken in pieces or 1 large lamb shank
- 3 medium onions, diced
- 1 tbsp of turmeric
- 1 tbsp flour
- 2 tbsp pearl barley
- Salt and black pepper as desired

Method

Add the bone marrow or lamb shank to a large pot and cover with cold water on a medium heat. When the water starts boiling, drain the water and return the pot to the heat. Add onion, turmeric and cover with water again. Add barley and chickpeas and leave on a low–medium heat for 3 hours.

If using bone marrow, when water is reduced to one third of the pot, take the bone marrow out.

In small bowl, add 5 spoons of water to flour and mix well. When you get to a smooth texture, add to the soup and mix well. Add salt and pepper.

Continue to cook on a low heat for 30 more minutes until you get to a runny soup.

In case it's cooked for a recovering patient with lamb shank, it is said it's better not to give the patient the meat – just the soup is good enough to bring back their strength.

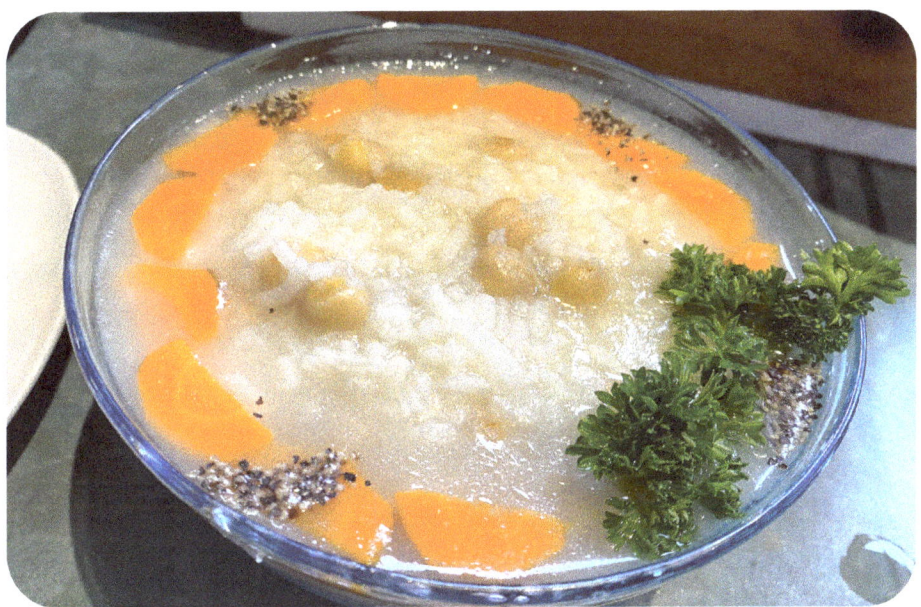

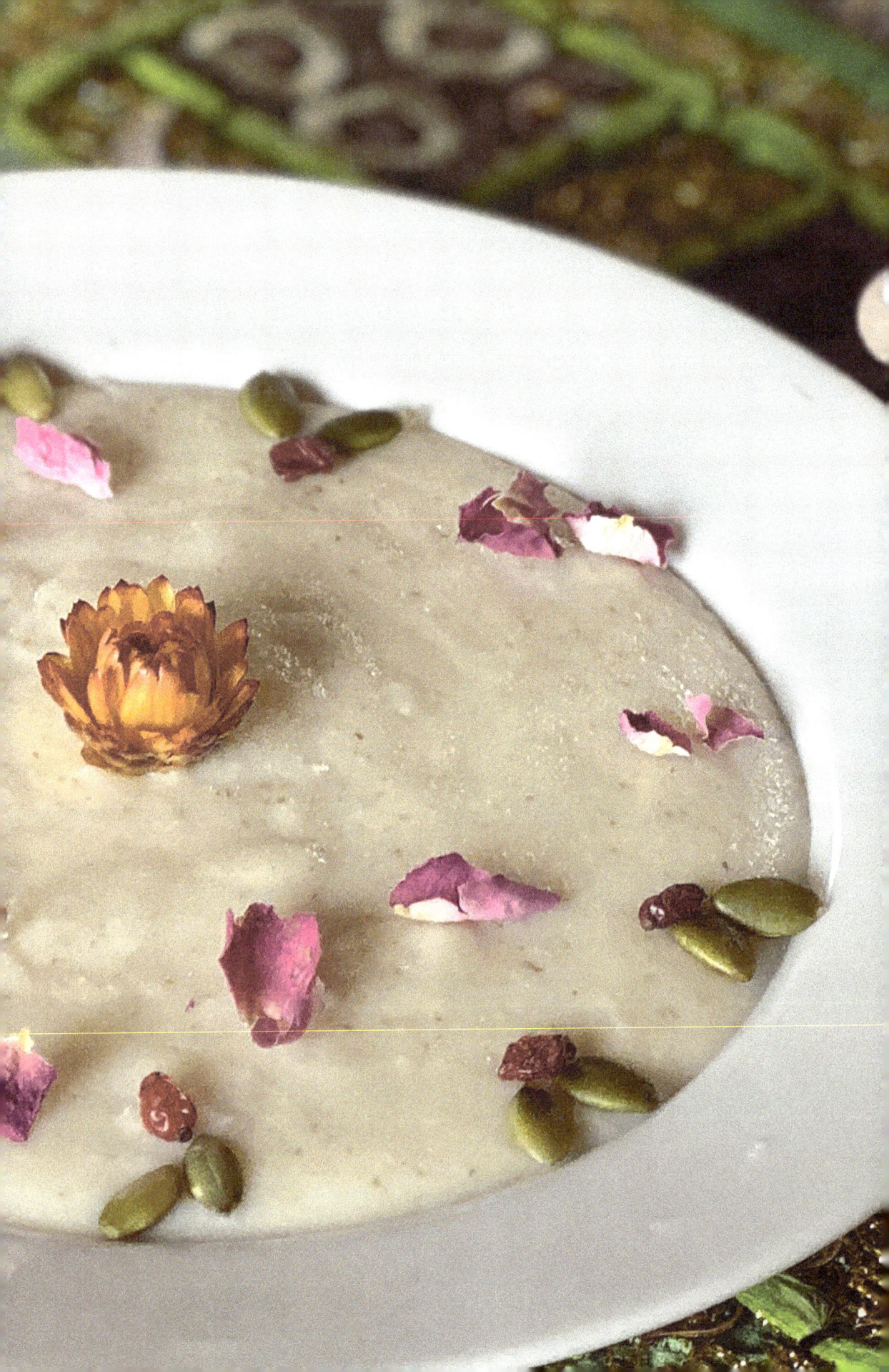

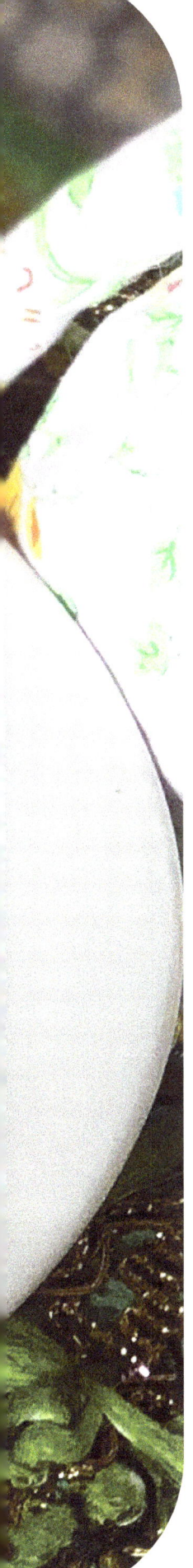

Harireh badam (silky almond meal)

Again, I don't really know whether to call this a dessert, medicine or food. But it's definitely the number one choice for babies first food after their mum's breast milk. Also people who are experiencing problems with their digestion are recommended to have this food at least once a week.

Being light to digest, it's also good option for the holy fasting month – if this falls in summer, sometimes people don't eat for 14–16 hours. After such long fast, you need to start with a light food.

The hero ingredient of this dish is almond powder. Although it's super easy to prepare, bringing the almond to the right place needs a bit of time. So it's not kind of food you suddenly decide to cook and then the next minute it will be on the table.

1/2 cup almond meal
1 glass milk
3 1/2 tablespoons sugar
1 tbsp rice flour or corn starch
1 tbsp rose water

Method

Add milk, sugar, corn starch or rice flour, and almond meal to a small pot over a low heat.

Do not let the mixture get too thick – you are aiming for a smooth and soft texture.

When the texture is right, add rosewater and stir for 10 seconds before taking off the heat.

If serving for dessert, garnish with dried rose petals and slivered pistachios.

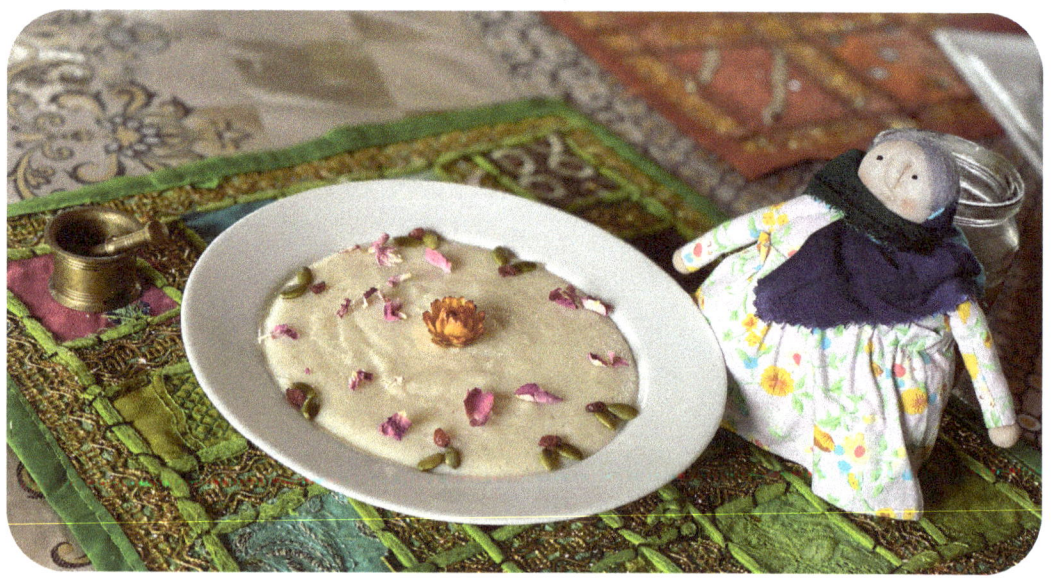

Food for weddings and formal ceremonies

Not long ago in Iran, nearly 40 years ago, most marriages were arranged marriages. You could hardly find two families that would agree on both sides to have a relationship before their marriage. Even if a boy and girl were brave enough to be friends before their marriage, their parents or other friends and relatives definitely didn't know anything about their relationship. Nowadays, everything is changed and parents and families look at marriage from a more open minded perspective.

Before, if a boy's parents wanted to find a proper wife for their son, they used to ask friends, family members or even people who were running businesses in their neighbourhood if they know a good girl. Some were lucky to find a proper future daughter-in-law among their family members and some needed to put in more effort on this task – usually, it was women's job to find a proper girl to their own family's standard.

In those days, women would go to religious ceremonies only open to women, and it was there that they would usually to find their son's future bride.

Then, – in case the two families were not already familiar with each other as friends or family –the courtship ceremony would start: it was time for both families to meet each other.

First, the groom's family would come to meet the bride family in the father of the bride's house. Usually, one or two older relatives like aunts will accompany the groom, along with his mother and sister. The male members of the groom's family would not be present in this meeting.

Then, if both families were happy to continue and if both families were open minded, they would let the groom and bride talk to each other in a separate room (in villages, the groom and bride would only have a chance to meet each other for the first time at their wedding ceremony). Then, the older family members took responsibility for the rest of the ceremony. They would set a date for the wedding day, usually this was on the date of one of the religious ceremonies.

Before the marriage ceremony, the groom and bride would go for their first shopping trip together. Again, in the older days, a few close family members would accompany them. The groom would buy gifts for his escorts too, and how many gifts the groom bought for his escorting group refers to his generosity and his financial situation but for each one he at least buys one gift, and a lot more for his bride.

These days, people are following more and more western customs and the bride and groom will go for wedding shopping all by themselves and with hardly anyone to accompany them. Even still, though no one is with them, they will buy a few gifts for the mother of both sides. All of these gifts should be beautifully wrapped and on the early morning of the wedding day, they will be sent to the bride's parents' house.

In the old days there was a special occupation just for this action. People in this occupation used to be called Tabgh (big either wooden or copper tray) Kesh (carrying). They normally worked in groups of seven people since seven is the lucky number in Persian culture. They would put all the wrapped gifts on their trays and follow each other to deliver all of the gifts from the groom's house to the bride's parents house, singing special wedding songs all the way. The wages for this job were paid by the bride's family as they were the one receiving the gifts. This was a very popular job and these men were busy through the whole year, except for the two holy months when there were no weddings.

On the morning before the marriage day, close members of both sides of the family will escort the groom and bride to their wedding bath. People accompanying the groom or bride in the bath would also sing and dance, as in those days, bathhouses were public, with a big entrance with single lockers for each visitor all around the room.

At the front door, there was usually someone sitting as supervisor – the supervisor's sex would depend on whether it was the men's or women's bath. He or she was responsible for charging visitors and reminding them of the rules in the public bath.

There were also always people available to give visitors traditional massage. It was believed that this traditional massage could fix lots of health issues. On the day of the wedding bath, both men and women would have separate wedding bath ceremonies.

Before the groom and bride and their accompanying guests arrived, a few people would bring gifts and food, sweets and soft drinks from the groom's house for the bride, and vice versa. The groom and bride would each arrive separately with their accompanying guests, and at their arrival, everyone in the public bath would start singing and dancing.

Each of their parents would also give gifts, which was usually money, to the bath servants. When the bath ceremonies were finished, everyone would go to the bride's house for the Henna party.

Henna parties used to be held separately: one for men in the groom's father house and one for only women in the bride's parents' house. Because of the religious government currently ruling in Iran they still have to have such ceremonies separately, but some families risk mixing their guest.

The night after the Henna party is the big wedding day. This is usually held in two ceremonies: First, an aisle part which is called Aghed. This is when very close relatives gather and a cleric who is authorised to do formal paper work recite and take both signatures and paperwork. On that day a special table with a mirror is set in front of the bride and groom, with candle holders on both sides of the mirror. Four young girls hold a piece of clean white fabric on top of the bride's head while another girl rubs two big sugar cubes onto the fabric, which is a sign of sweetness in their future life. The cleric will ask the bride whether she accepts this man as her husband, but the bride never says yes until the third time. Each time, the cleric reminds the bride of the gifts and conditions of the groom, and finally after the third time, the bride asks the permission of her parents and then says yes. Once she has said yes, the groom's mother should give her a piece of gold as her first gift, and then all close relatives respectively give her their gifts which are either gold or cash. Then, it's time for the second part of the ceremony, the reception where all the other guest are invited too.

Guests are served with fruits, sweets and soft drinks and in some states, like Azarbayjan and Tabriz, with good quality nuts too.

Food served at weddings used to be limited to one or two dishes but these days, a huge variety of very colourful food and desserts from Persian and international menus is served.

At the end of the night, a caravan of close relatives escort the bride and groom to their new home. All the furniture in their new home, which is called Jahaz, is usually provided by the bride's parents. The more luxurious the Jahaz, the more credit is given to the bride and her family by the groom's relatives.

Although the variety of wedding food is so wide, there are a few dishes that are the star of every wedding dinner table, and these are the recipes I share with you here.

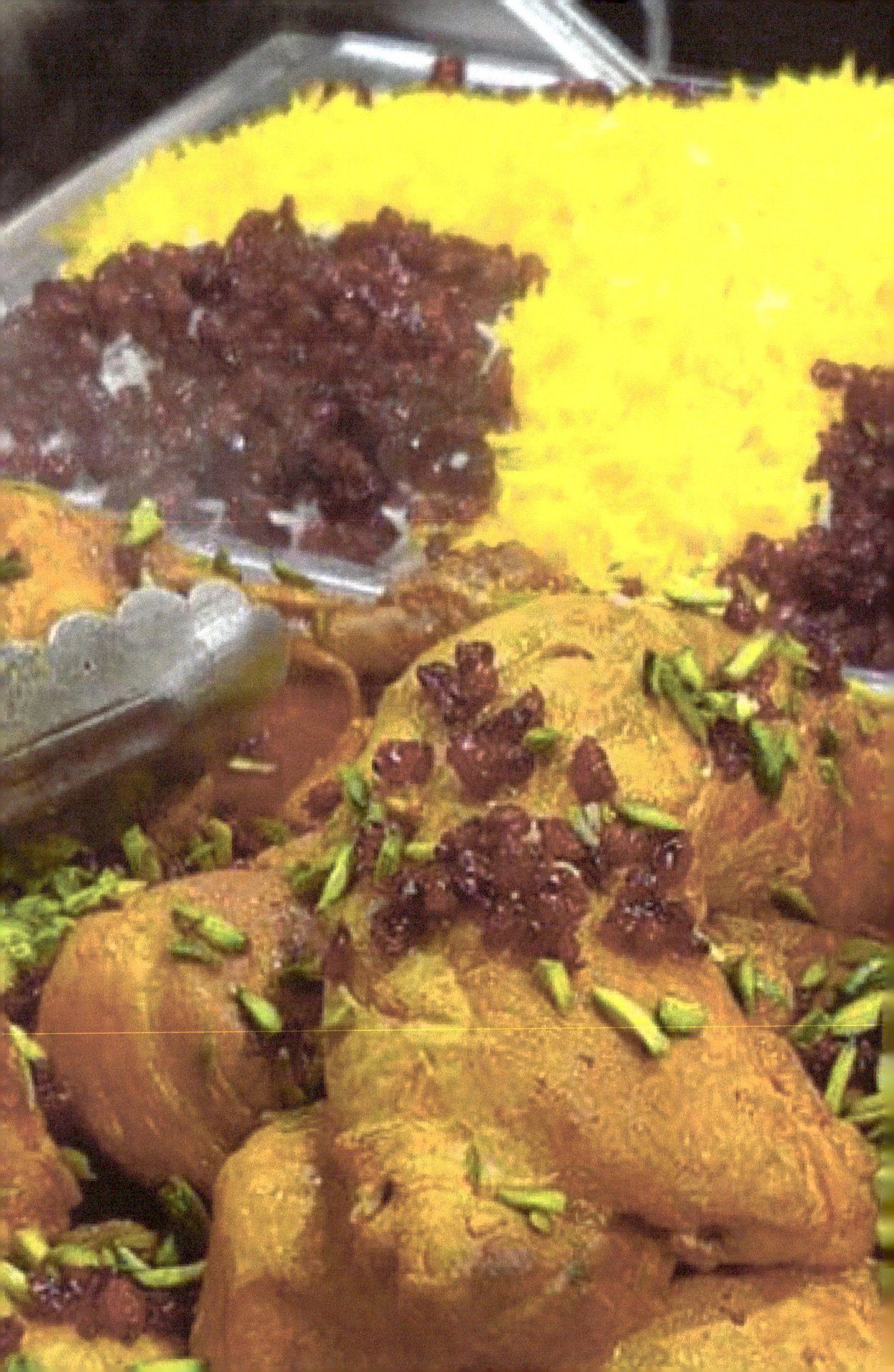

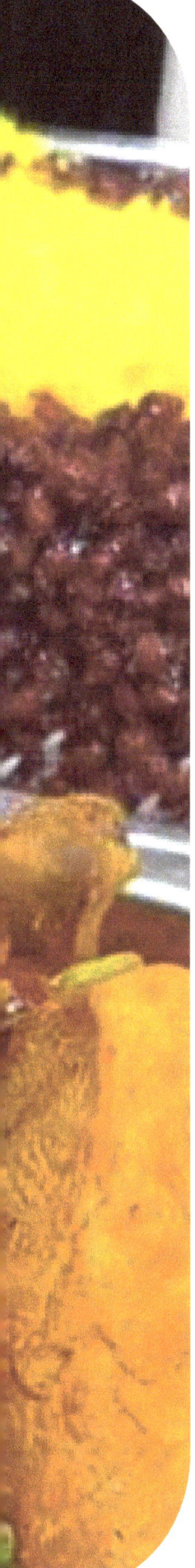

Zereshk Polo Morgh

(chicken barberry and saffron rice)

Although this food is very common among Iranians, it is always served at Iranian weddings.

Barberries used to grow wild in the north east states, especially in Khoorasan. where the best saffron is grown too. Now, barberries are cultivated in other states as well since there is high demand for this product all over the country.

When I put barberries in some of my dishes, I see many western style cook mistake them for pomegranate seeds, as they look similar, with almost the same taste but they are way different in usage and availability – since barberries are dry seeds available all year round but fresh pomegranate seeds are only available in autumn and used in limited foods.

Although this is a formal food, it is also very easy to cook. If you have a friend coming over unexpectedly, and you're anxious to serve them with good food, this could be a good choice as it could be ready to eat in less time that is needed to prepare and cook other luxurious foods. This is a very popular dish – the different taste of barberries makes you go for it.

Serves 4

Prep and cooking time: 45 minutes

- 1 piece of chicken, either leg or breast according to your preference, per serve
- 1 plate cooked rice per serve
- 1 1/2 tsp saffron
- 3 tbsp barberries per serve
- 1 tbsp sugar
- 1 tbsp salt
- 1/2 tbsp slivered pistachios (optional)
- 2 tbsp butter
- Oil, for frying chicken
- 1 large onion

Method

Follow the method provided in earlier recipes to cook your rice.

Wash chicken and fry in oil on each side till you get a bit of colour. Roughly slice and transfer to pot with one of glass of water and half of tablespoon of salt. Cook on a low heat until the chicken is soft. Drain the chicken and reserve the sauce to serve.

Wash and drain the barberries.

Brew the saffron with ice or hot boiling water as explained in earlier recipes and set aside.

Melt butter in a separate pan. Add barberries, brewed saffron and sugar and fry for 10 seconds. Do not fry any longer since barberries burn fast.

To prepare to dish up, take three full tablespoons of plain rice and mix with the barberry mixture, gently mix and set aside.

To dish up, first put plain rice on the plate. Gently place the chicken on the rice and top with the saffron barberry rice and the rest of the barberry mixture. Serve hot, with the sauce separately.

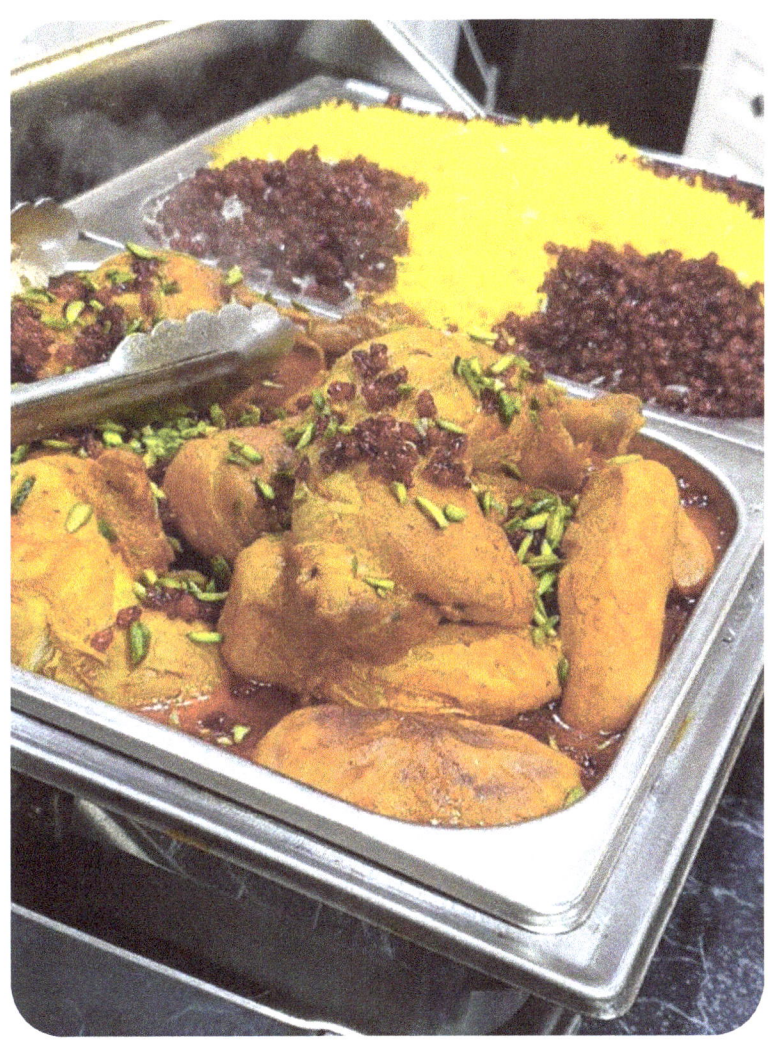

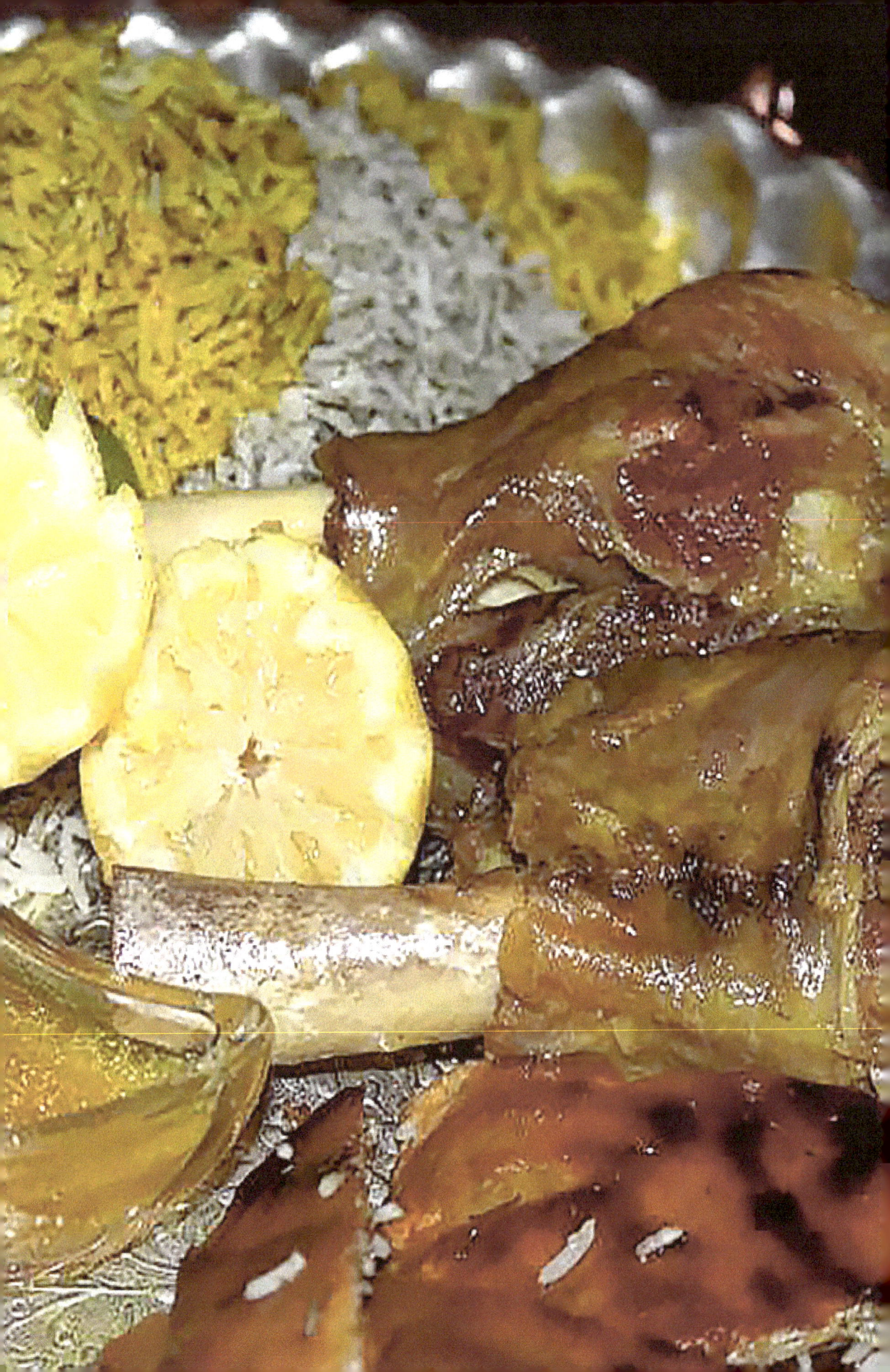

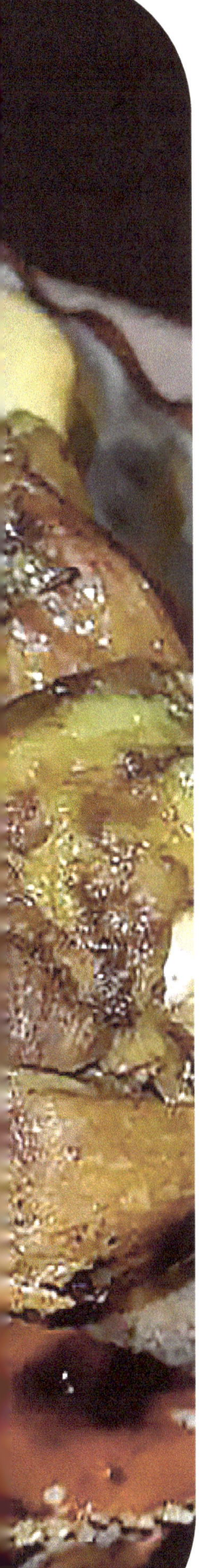

Baghali Polo
(Lamb shank with rice and broad beans and dill)

Baghali Polo is one of the most luxurious Persian foods and by far one of most popular Persian dishes on restaurant menus. It's another dish that is always available in any formal ceremony, especially at weddings.

It could be served by chicken instead of lamb, but lamb shank is more popular. Besides, it's hardly served with chicken at weddings as the other wedding popular dish already has chicken in it. In some ceremonies, they cook the broad bean and rice and serve with both cooked lamb shank and chicken separately so you can choose between them.

This dish reputation goes back to the Safavi dynasty, though its origin is not clear and it's now very common in all states. The magical combination between lamb shank and rice with purified butter has made this a favourite among tourists –

anyone who has visited Iran will remember this food as one of their best memories during their journey.

There are two types of broad beans to cook for this dish: Fresh, which are only available at some special times of the year, or frozen. The best taste for this dish comes from using fresh broad beans with fresh chopped dill and Persian aromatic rice with ghee on top.

So when the market is full with fresh broad beans people buy large amounts, in some families, over 100 kilograms. First, because they use a lot throughout the year and second, because after removing the first hard pods and then the second skins too, the large amount comes to almost a third of the original amount. These days, they are usually preserved in freezers but it is also still common to dry them as well. If using the second option, they always dry the broad beans in the shade.

This is because if they are sundried, their colour will change to yellow, which makes them inappropriate to use in formal Baghali Polo. Although the yellow dried broad beans are still good for a simple basic version with turmeric and rice.

For lamb shank:

Serves 6

Prep and cooking time: 1 hour 45 minutes

- 6 lamb shanks, one per serve
- 1 1/2 large onions, finely chopped
- 4 cloves garlic
- 1/2 tbsp turmeric
- 2 bay leaves
- 1 tsp pepper
- 2 tbsp brewed saffron
- 3 tablespoons oil
- 1/2 tbsp salt
- 1/4 cup lemon juice

Method

Wash lamb shanks. Heat oil in a large pan and fry each lamb shank slightly on both sides.

Add onion, garlic, turmeric and bay leaves.

Add water to cover the lamb shanks and cook on a low to medium heat for one hour, until soft.

When the lamb shanks are soft, add salt and lemon juice and continue to cook on a low heat until the extra liquid is vaporised but not totally reduced.

For rice and fava broad beans:

Serves 6

Prep time: 15 min

Cooking time: 45 min

- 4 cups long grain basmati rice, washed and soaked with 2 tbsp at least 2 hours in advance
- 3 cups fresh or frozen broad beans, double shelled
- 1/3 cup vegetable oil
- 1/3 tsp ground turmeric
- 1 tsp ground cinnamon
- 50 grams butter or ghee
- 2 tbsp brewed-saffron
- 3 bunches fresh dill, washed and chopped or 200 grams of dried dill
- 1 piece flatbread or one potato, thinly sliced

Method

Bring one third of a large pot of water to the boil.

Once water is boiling, add soaked rice and turmeric. When the mixture starts boiling, check the grains of rice. When the outer layer of the grain is soft but still hard inside, it's time to drain in a colander. Rinse with cold water.

In another, pot add double shelled broad beans until half cooked (be careful not to cook them too soft). Drain and set aside.

Add three tablespoons of vegetable oil to a deep, medium pot and cover with one layer of flatbread or thin slices of potato.

Add rice, broad beans and dill in layers.

Push the rice from the sides of the pot into the shape of a mountain peak. Make a big hole in the middle to steam. Add butter and cinnamon on top.

Wrap the lid of the pot with a clean tea towel and leave it on the pot so all sides are tightly covered with the tea towel.

Cook on a medium-high heat for 10 minutes and then on a low heat for a further 35 minutes.

After 45 minutes, take the rice off the heat and dish up onto plates. Serve one cooked lamb shank on each side of each plate.

Serve the extra sauce from the lamb shanks in a separate bowl.

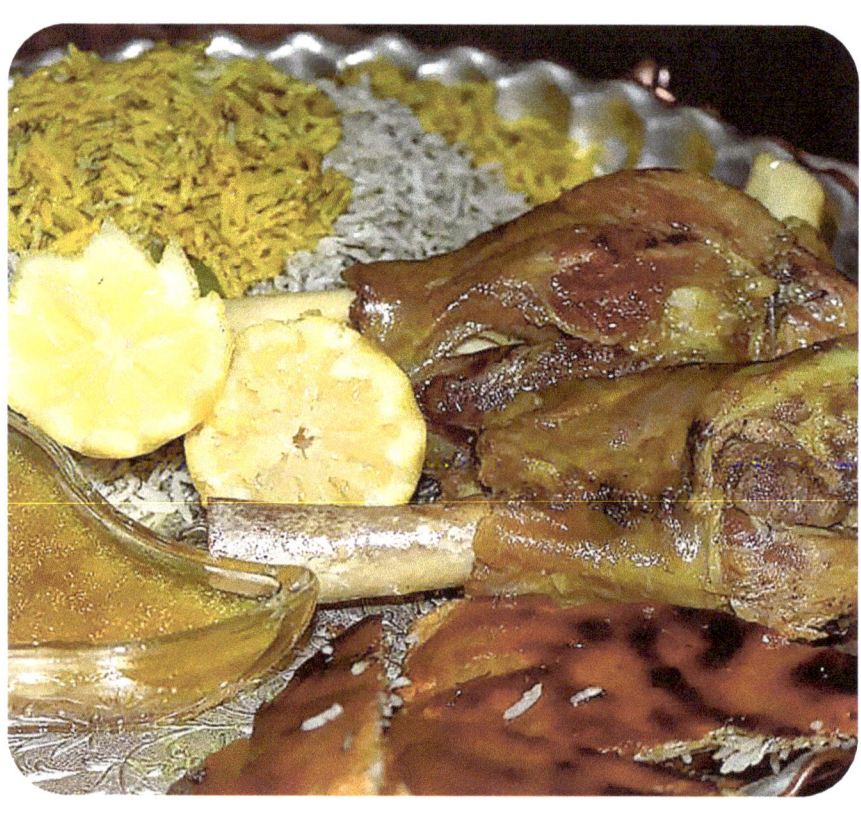

Food for weddings and formal ceremonies

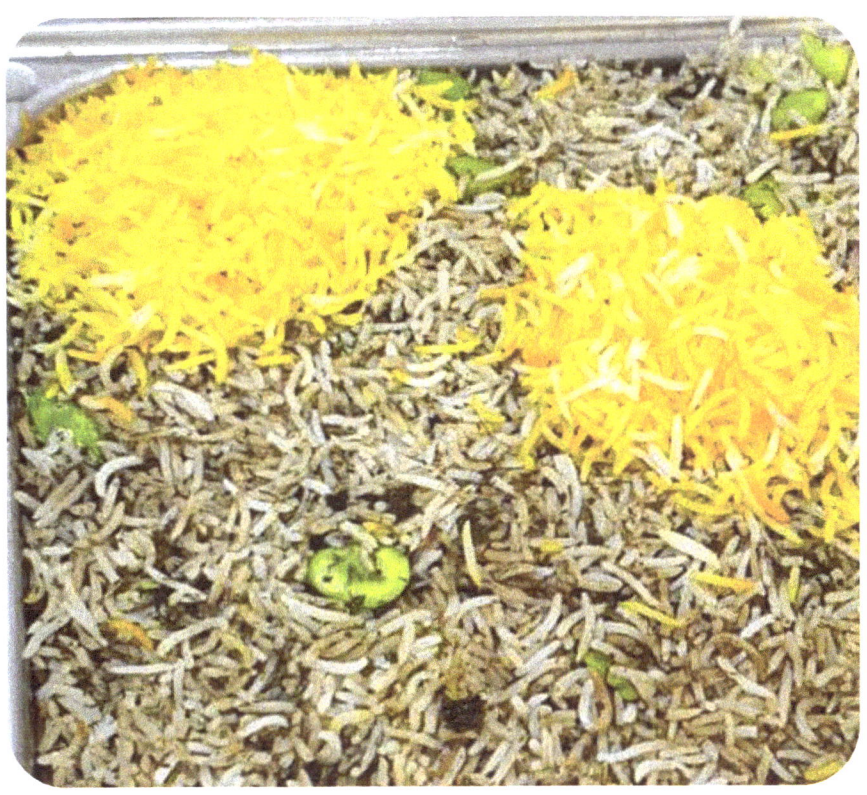

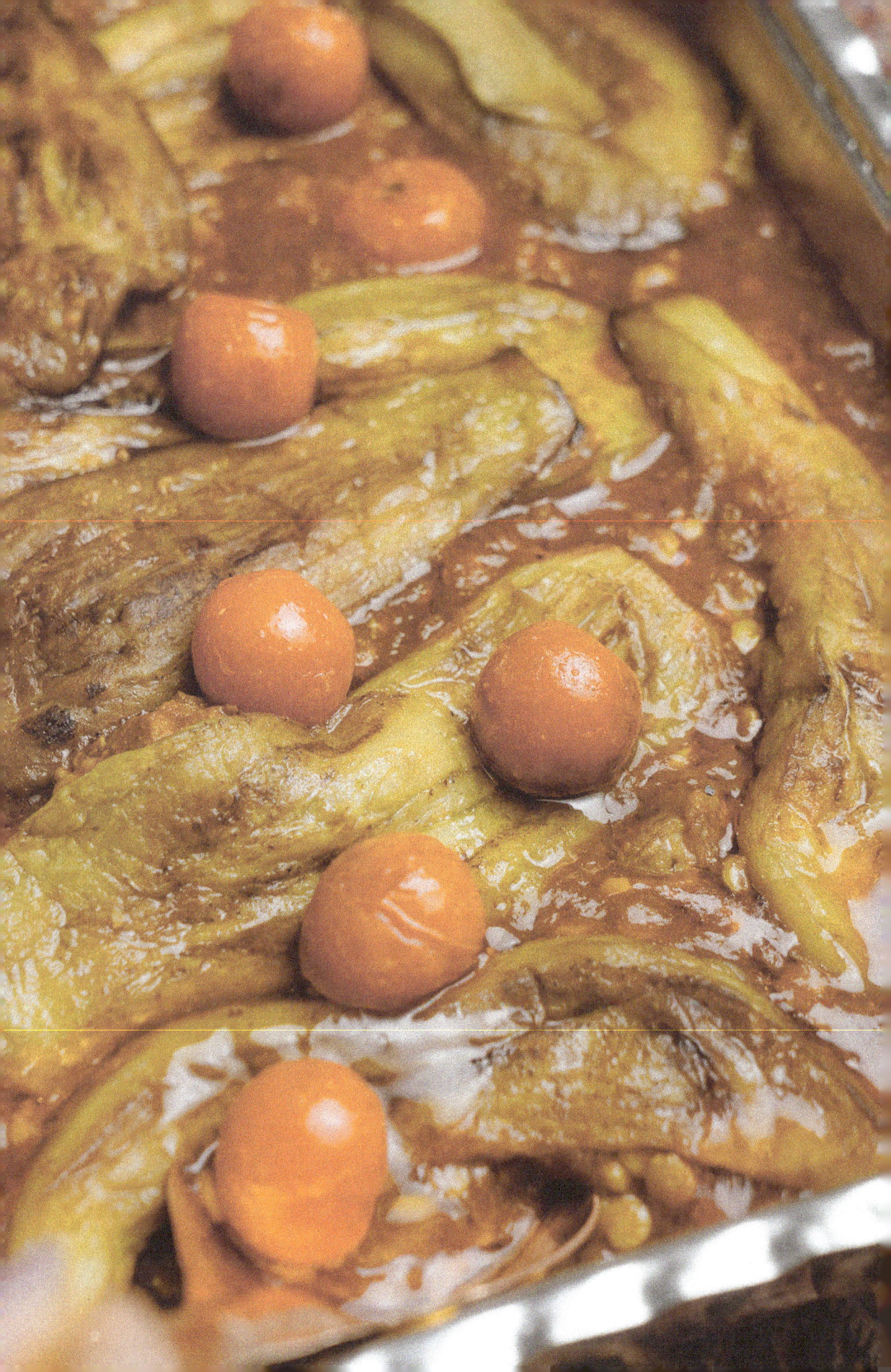

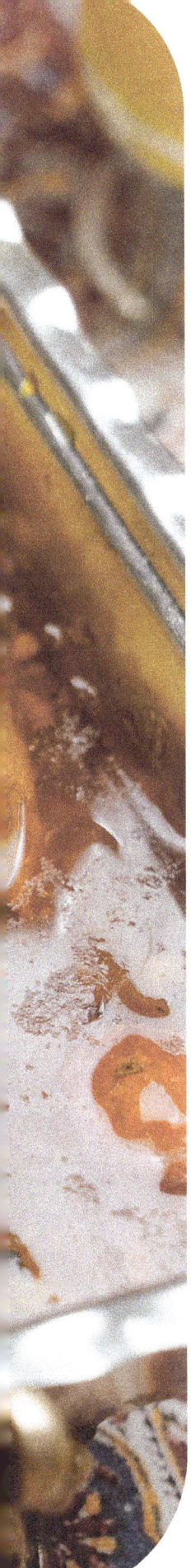

Gheymeh & Ghoormeh

Although these two each are a separate and totally different persian stew with completely different cooking process and taste, but in times of giving expression of a well served guest they use these together like they say oh well done ! You have been served Gheymeh and Ghoormeh.

Also these twin words which each one points to one of most known persian stew sometimes are used together and it's when Iranian are giving expression of having very luxury food for a guest.

Now a days all sort of western style food are considered to be known as luxurious food in Iran. But in old days when someone was using these two together first thing came to your mind was you knew the cook has put a lot of effort in serving you and second you knew your gonna get two of most well known yet delicious stew.

Gheymeh and Ghoormeh: Gheymeh in vocabulary means small pieces of meat.

Mainly use lamb meat but it's possible to cook with lamb however cooking Gheymeh with lamb is more delicious since it's get its real taste from fat in meat and lamb is more fatty. By the time of cook this stew lamb meat should be cut in small pieces with little bite of fat in each piece.

It's reputation in Iranian cuisine refers to thousands years ago and it always was one of the most common food served in king court in very old days.

After Arabs invaded Iran and Iranian accepted Islam as their religion in the country it also became one of the main food being served in religious ceremonies. Any kind of food served in religious ceremonies is called Nazri.

Nazr which is still very common among Iranian is people make a deal with God in their heat that if their wishes come true they do any special service to the community. Most of the time this Nazri service to community delivers by distributing food among people.

There are some holy months or days in Iranian calendar and during those times you see people distributing food among strangers in the streets. Gheymeh is very common Nazri food.

There are two different kind of Gheymeh one is served with thin slices of fried potato on top of the stew and the second kind with exactly same ingredients and same cooking process is served by thin lengths slices of fried eggplant.

To be honest I never been able to choose which kind is better because both are so tasty and delicious but for serving as Nazri the one with fried potato is more common which is called Gheymeh Nazri. Although Gheymeh Nazri is not different with normal Gheymeh in cooking process or ingredients people believe when it's cooked for Nazri process it's more delicious and they believe the spirit and energy behind that religious reason to cook Gheymeh makes it unique in taste and more delicious. Yellow split lentil is the supporting actor this dish while leading actor is small piece of lamb meat with tiny bit of fat in each piece, other ingredients which their role in processing a delicious Gheymeh are also very important are spices, golden fried onion, tomato paste , dried lemon. Spices in Persian foods are used but most of the time not so much heat in our food, turmeric and and beautiful flavour and aroma of saffron big yes and always.

To bring out that real flavour of of Persia of we add rose water few minutes before serving, I think rosewater is the reason people think Gheymeh Nazri is different with other Gheymeh cooked for daily taking as Gheymeh Nazri has always rosewater but in normal cooking sometimes they skip adding rosewater in last stage.

The reason that rose water is added to stew in very last minute is the secret how to save the flavour of rose water since in case rose water is boiled it will lose its unique aroma. Gheymeh with fried eggplant as I said is very common but more used in daily menu and less for Nazri.

The variety of eggplant dishes in different states of Iran is so huge you can almost say Iranian don't just eat eggplants they are deeply in love with it. Iranian believe the food they serve in religious ceremonies must be from best quality. They also believe they must offer their best to their holy profits otherwise is being disrespectful to their holy profit. It always is served with saffron rice and of course no Persian stew is complete without saffron jewelled rice and special Persian sides like freshly cut herbs or yogurt and mint and cucumber dip.

Gheymeh with fried potato or with fried eggplant

Serving : 4

Prep time: 30 min

Cooking : 1 h / 30 min

Total : 2 h

- Lamb leg 500 grams
- Yellow split lentil 1 and half medium size cup
- 2 large potato for Gheymeh with fried potato washed, thin sliced in length and deep fried

Or

- 1 large eggplant in case for Gheymeh with eggplant peeled and thin sliced in length and fried in both sides
- 1 large onion
- 3 dried lemon (could be fined in Persian shops if not available replace with two table spoon of lemon juice)
- 3 table spoon of tomato paste
- 1/2 cup of vegetable oil if potato or eggplant are fried separately otherwise 1 cup of vegetable oil
- 1 cinnamon stick

- 2 tsp of tumeric
- 1/2 tsp of black pepper
- Salt as desired
- Rosewater 2 tablespoons

Method

Finely chop onion. Cut lamb in small cubes ideally with a bite of fat in each piece. If your lamb is with bones keep the bone to cook in stew for extra flavour.

With 4 table spoon of oil in a frying pan fry lamb cubes to brown in each side and when fried transfer to a medium size pot.

Add fine chopped onion to meat in the pot, 1 table spoon vegetable oil and put on medium heat and stir regularly for about 10 minutes.

Add tomato paste and stir and let all ingredients in pot combine together for 4 more minutes, add turmeric, black pepper and give one more stir.

Add two cups of boiling water, stir to combine and then reduce the heat to low temperature.

Poke dried lemon with a fork so the stew can absorb their flavour and add to the pot (if couldn't find dry lemon replace with lemon juice but add lemon juice 15 minutes before serving).

In separate pot wash and add 2 cups of boiling water with yellow split lentil until it's soft but not mushy.

Once cooked rinse with cold water and add to stew when meat is soft and cooked and stew is getting thick.

It's important to add cooked lentil in almost last stage of cooking process otherwise lentil will be over cooked and starts getting mushy.

Meat also should be cooked on medium to low heat for 1 hour before adding cooked lentil.

While cooking the meat check if it has enough water if not only add hot boiling water, never add cold water to stew that will kill the flavour.

Once the meat is cooked and tender, take the cinnamon stick out and add lentil, in very last stage for stew add two tablespoons of rosewater.

Do not let the rosewater boil, boiling will kill the flavour of rosewater.

Preap for frying chips of eggplant.

Wash, and cut potatoes in length in thin sizes.

Wash again add salt and dry.

In small pan deep fry the potato like any normal chips and once you get enough golden colour and felt the crunch take potatoes out and leave them on a paper towel to take out that extra oil.

When stew is thick enough pour in serving plate with fried chips on top and serve with saffron basmati rice.

If you want to serve with fried eggplant:

Wash, peel and cut the eggplant in length and medium thin size, dry with paper towel and brush each side with yogurt. Brushing with yogurt is for absorbing less oil.

Once you get that golden fried colour from eggplant leave them on paper towel again serve on top of the stew and Noosh E Jan.

(Bonna petit in Persian.)

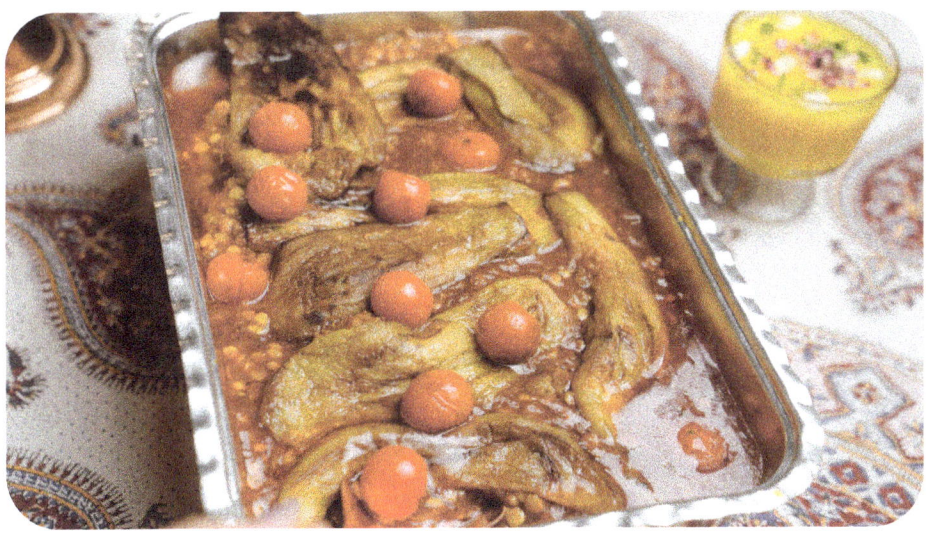

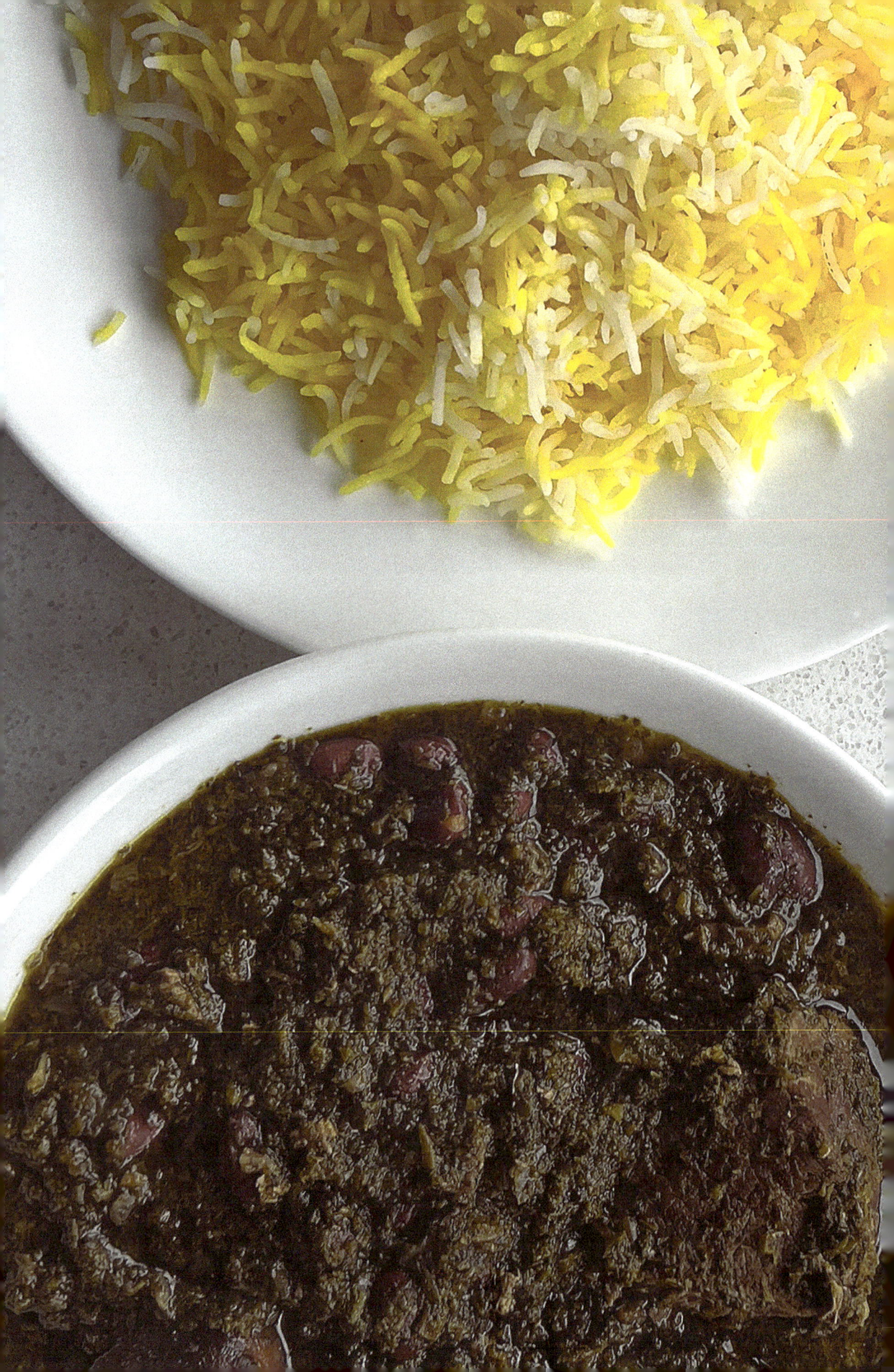

Ghoormeh Sabzi
a classic traditional lamb and herb stew

I'm not exaggerating if I call Ghoormeh Sabzi as most well known and most favourite Persian food among Iranians.

It's the only Persian food that world international heritage has registered it as national heritage for Iranians.

Iranians are so much in love with Ghoormeh Sabzi they have a national day in their calendar as Ghoormeh Sabzi national day and it's first Saturday in November (Azar as Iranian calendar). It's a very big delicious day for Iranian and its only 3 days after thanksgiving day in America.

It has been in Iranian foods for such long time almost no one knows to when its reputation refers too or which state is the origin.

Few other countries which share borders with Iran also have this food on their national cuisine menu and that proves it has long reputation as all these countries like Afghanistan, Azerbaija, Armenian, Pakistan. All for all have been part of the Iranian empire centuries ago and the Iran empire was ruling on them for centuries.

Some believe its reputation refers to more than 5 thousands years ago by paying attention to its ingredients and cooking process it might be true as all the ingredients are and have been very accessible in Iran forever.

Noticing it's name it has two syllables: Ghoormeh and Sabzi

Name contains two syllables and there is a reason for that.

Ghoormeh means small pieces of meat cut with knife and had been prepared with special process as I will describe here and Sabzi means herb. In some states it's called herb stew although there are many other dishes with herb as hero ingredient but everyone knows for this herb stew it refers to same Ghoormeh Sabzi. In very old days there was no cooling system to keep food fresh in hot season and in the other hand it was not easy and in some cases impossible to provide some of the ingredients for cooking as they were out of season in cold month of the years.

Transportation system also was very limited to animals .

In such situations it was not easy to provide ingredients for daily use. People had their own ways to preserve foods for their essentials and daily use. One of these ways was salting to profit meat and mainly it was lamb meat.

In last month of every summer which sheep had reasonable price they use to buy and preserve it in salt in large containers made from clay and then seal it with clay or cement. Once it was sealed no one was allowed to open it before winter, during year every time they wanted to cook meaty food they used to open those containers and take as their usage.

Although in very old days people used to eat simple food most of the time but for any special occasions or even for celebrating weekends with family members or by the time any guests would arrive unexpectedly, which they should have good and sometimes formal food, they simply had that preserved meat with any other fresh and available sides.

These preserved meat Ghoormeh didn't need any time to be cooked and it was ready to add to any other ingredients or flavour to make dish out of it or to be eaten as it was with any other side or simply with bread.

Even considering nutritional benefits of a food you can say Ghoormeh Sabzi has all required factors to be called a completely nutritional food as the ingredients such as meat, beans , herbs are all main factors of food pyramid to complete daily need for food are in it. Because of herbs being involved as main ingredients many think it's origin is North of Iran because as I said earlier North of Iran is more green than any other state in Iran but the reality is its not obviously clear where is real origin of this King of Persian food Ghoormeh Sabzi. It might not be as common as Gheymeh in occasional and National ceremonies but because almost everyone all over the country is so much in love with this food you definitely will see it being served in many occasions either for national or religious ceremonies.

For Zartostian who are in minority in the Iranian community it is a must to serve Ghoormeh Sabzi in first day of the year to their family members. There is a saying among Persian people as a cook is a good cook when they can cook a good and well accomplished Ghoormeh Sabzi.

I remember when someone with great cooking talent was defined well by others, they will answer back well we should taste her Ghoormeh Sabzi to judge about how good she is her cooking. Whatever I say or any words I give you about this dish you may not be able to define what is Ghoormeh Sabzi real place in Persian people life and how important is this dish to Iranian it's not just a delicious food to them it's some how their valued identity.

For those who have tried it Once you have it it's hard to forget. It's very unique aroma is mesmerising and taste of that green and dark herb gravy with sour taste will penetrate to the depth of your mind. Many believe when you finished cooking Ghoormeh Sabzi you shouldn't eat it straight away, leave it in the fridge and eat it the next day.

I don't know why but they are right, it's really taste better after being left for one day in fridge and reheated.

There is actually a proverb made based on this, when they want to give compliment to a middle age woman that how young she looks they say oh God she is like a Ghoormeh Sabzi left one night in fridge which means she even looks better than her young age.

Serving: 4

Preap : 30 min

Time to cook : 4 hours on very low heat

- 500 lamb shoulder cut in cubes better to have fat in each cube
- 1/3 cup red kidney beans
- (if use can bean 1 can is enough but remember to add can beans when meat is cooked well)
- 1 cup vegetable oil

- 1 large onion finely chopped
- 1 bunch parsley
- 1 bunch coriander
- 1 bunch chives
- 1/2 bunch spinach
- 1 flat tablespoons of dried fenugreek
- 3 Persian dried lemon (if not available add 2 extra tablespoons of lemon juice to the stew at last stage by time of serving)
- 1 teaspoon of crumbled saffron threads
- 2 tablespoons of lemon juice (add in last stage of cooking, in case you can't find Persian dried lemon)
- Salt as desired just also remember to add salt when meat is well cooked, otherwise cooking process will even be longer.

For Ghoormeh Sabzi it should always be served with plain cooked rice ideally with saffron rice.

Long grain basmati rice is always best choice for any different Persian dish contains rice except for Persian soups or Persian desserts contain rice for those dish always try broken rice (rice which are in small grain size).

Method

Wash all the herbs and leave on a drainage to drop out extra water.

Start chopping all the herbs very finely on a cutting board , all herbs except dried fenugreek. Once all the herbs are very well and finely chopped transfer them to a medium size pan for frying and start to fry finely chopped herbs with two tablespoons of vegetable oil.

Following These two steps in having well cooked Ghoormeh Sabzi is very important.

Fry herbs until the fried herbs colour has changed to a dark green colour and set aside. In a medium size pan with medium to low heat ,add two tablespoons of oil, add cube size lambs meat, fry each side and when meat colour is about to change add finely chopped onion, stir and let to be on medium to low heat for more 7-10 minutes.

Add black pepper (optional, never add salt in this stage before meat is well cooked otherwise it takes longer for meat to be cooked).

If your using dry red kidney beans it's time to add it to the pot and if your using can red kidney beans save it for later when meat is well cooked and stew is start getting thick otherwise stew will be mushy if you add can kidney beans at the beginning of cooking process.

Add two glasses of boiling to the pot with fried herbs. Poke dried lemon and leave them in stew to drain out it's flavour in to the stew. Do not add replaced lemon juice in this stage if you don't have access to dried lemon, save it for later to add lemon juice when the stew is start getting thick and meat is cooked is good time to add lemon juice and can kidney beans.

Turn the heat down to medium low and let all ingredients marry and combine well together in the pot.

During cooking time whenever you felt water in stew is not enough add another glass of boiling water.

When meat is cooked and you feel enough thickness in the stew add your saffron, salt and finally add lemon juice if you prefer more sour taste add a bite more lemon juice, I personally prefer adding tamarind sauce with 1/2 teaspoons sumac but this is my option as I like more dominant sour taste in the stew. Enough thickness for stew usually happens after 4 hours on low heat.

In last stage fry dried fenugreek in two tablespoons of oil and add to the stew, let it on very low heat for 15 more minutes and then it's time to serve.

It could be served either plain cooked rice or ideally serve with saffron rice.

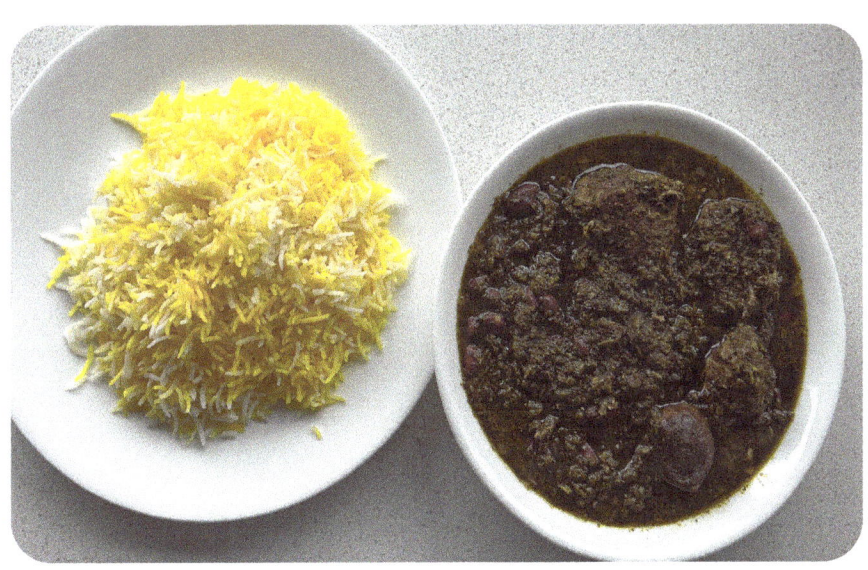

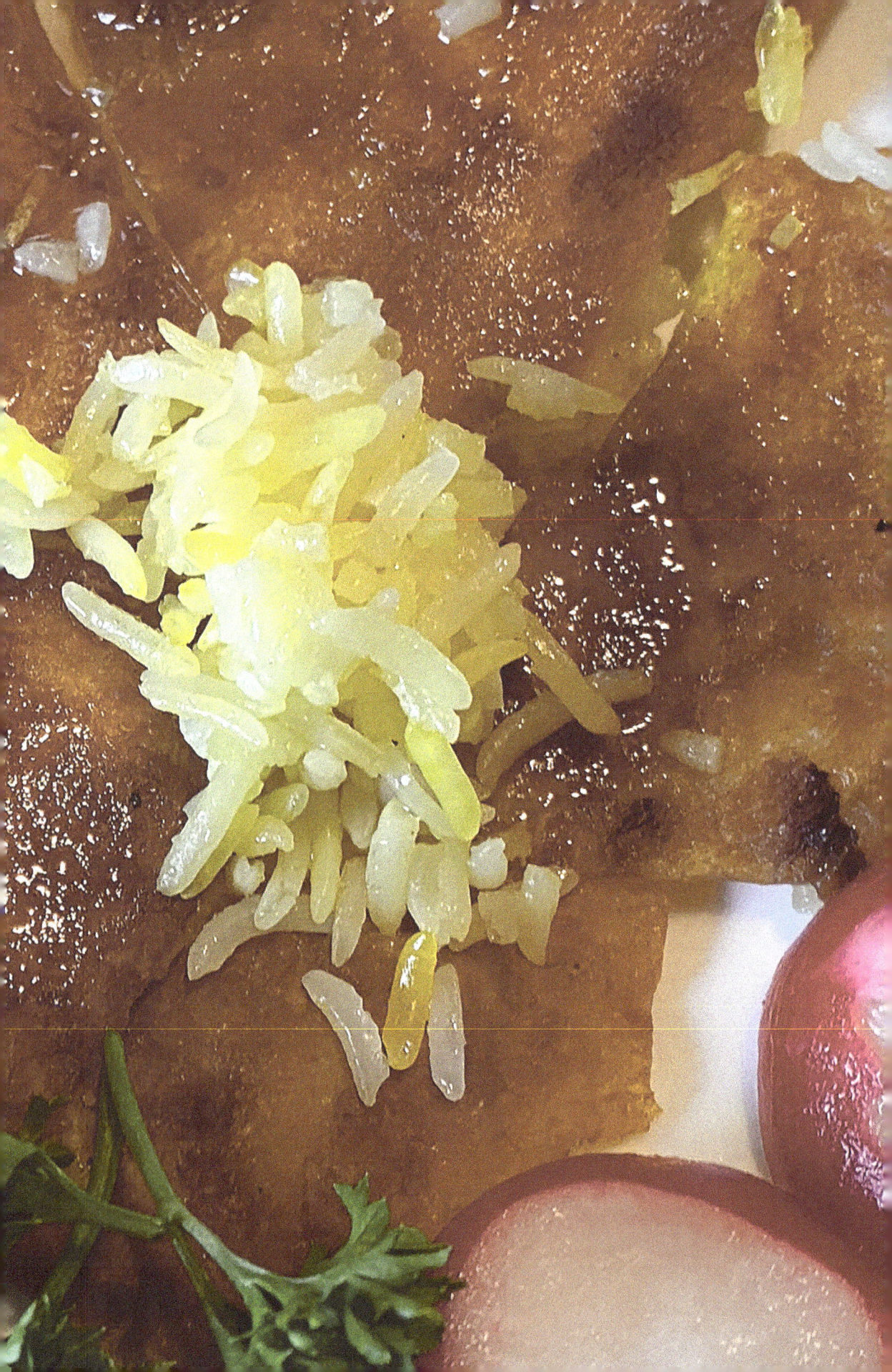

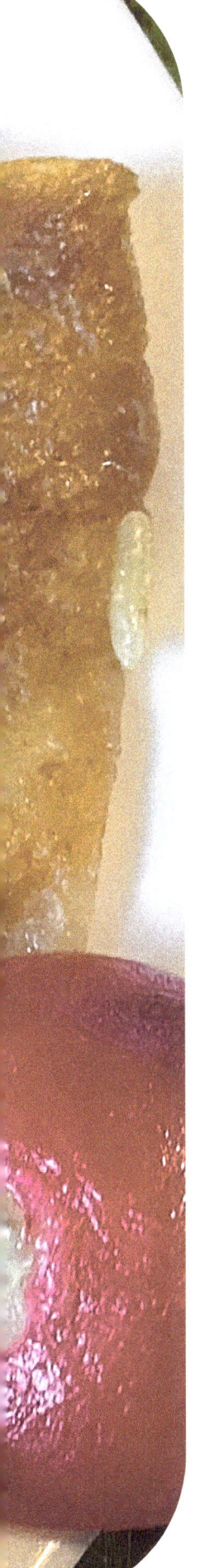

Tah-Dig and Tah-Chin

I really didn't know in which food section is best for Tah-Dig. Although I left it in kids favourite food section but in fact it is everyone else favourite including kids. It's a thin crust of slightly browned rice at the bottom of rice, super crunchy , super tasty however it's not always produced with rice and it's possible to make a good Tah-Dig out of other ingredients too , which later here will point to them.

Rice Tah–Dig is produced during cooking of rice over and by a very low direct heat from the flame. It's pleasant crunchy taste is something that almost no one can resist, that's why everyone on table always fighting over it. Best Tah–Dig is when it has that perfect golden crust in last layer at the bottom of the pot. Being very creative caused cooks inventing big variety of Tah–Dig made from thin layers of Lavash , thin layers of potato, beetroot, pumpkin, lettuce for rice and herbs, grated potato, rice with saffron mixed with yogurt and egg (called Tah-chin mostly served in formal event).

For Tah–Chin I will give your more information in another section), but the most popular one is rice itself, rice Tah–Dig. There is a saying among Iranian anyone who eats too much Tah–Dig will have a very wet and rainy wedding night, and who likes rainy wedding night.

This proverb was invented by clever parents who wanted to trick kids and stop them from having all Tah–Dig on the table since it's so tasty not only kids but also adults can't resist it too. Parents needed to come up with a solution so kids would let them have some Tah–Dig too otherwise kids would finish it all and leave no Tah–Dig for parents.

This was a clever proverb to trick some Tah–Dig lovers, but not all of them. After all who can resist from that buttery, saffron crunchy rice unless their worried for their rainy weeding night. For producing Tah–Dig you don't need a exact recipe just knowing few cooking hacks and being aware of when it's right time to lower down the heat while rice is cooking is enough . Following these hacks and steps will give you a perfect Tah–Dig.

Also knowing how to adjust the heat from medium to low while rice is cooking is the secret to perfect Tah–Dig and that comes only from experience. Iranian are famous for their hospitality and when a guest drops to a Persian house it's like everything in the house belongs to that guest but for Tah–Dig I doubt they give up on their share of Tah–Dig to please even their dear guest. If a guest is invited to a Persian house doesn't matter how big eater is the guest the food must be far more than he can finish it. That is a sign of respect, there should be a lots of left over when guest leaves the table.

It's possible for all kinds of Persian food except Tah(bottom) Dig(pot).Well doesnt matter how big is your rice pot there is never enough Tah–Dig for everyone on the table. It's so incredibly tasty and crunchy that people prefer to start with Tah - Dig rather than with anything else on the table. No one ever says No to Tah–Dig.

Maybe love of Tah–Dig leaded Iranian to invent Tah–Chin, the only Persian rice which Tah–Digey in every coroners. Tah–Chin is a Persian rice dish but it's Tah–Digey dish maybe by inventing this dish, everyone on table could have enough Tah–Dig and fight on the table for this delicious creature could be ended. But how Tah–Dig itself started getting so popular, Of course it always was there but it wasn't as popular as it is now. Like for every other food , there is also a story for Tah–Dig and how love for Tah–Dig have happened.

They say in very very old days. In One of Iranian King's court (they don't know which King) court chef always used to serve first and best part of rice to King and his guests and court people so only whatever was left in the bottom of pots part was for servants to eat. They were never allowed to eat before King and his guests which means fluffy and shiny parts of rice was served to them and lucky servants had to eat whatever left in bottom of pot, well they were lucky as they had lots of Tah–Dig to eat and King and others did t even know what is Tah–Dig. Servants were actually were very happy for this arrangements. One day when servants finished serving King and it was their turn to eat leftovers, there was not enough leftovers for all of them , they started fighting over Tah–Dig with making lots of noise.

King heard their noise and called the head chef and asked what is that noise why there is a fight in kitchen. Chef told him they are fighting over Tah–Dig, King didn't know what is Tah–Dig , he never had it, he always had top, which he thought is the best part of rice. He wanted to know what is it making servants to fighting over it, he ordered chef to bring him Tah–Dig and it was then when he found out what he has been missing all the time, he said : oh , it is best part of pot and servants had right to fight over it. Starting from then King fell in love with Tah–Dig and he ordered chef to bring him Tah–Dig first rather than serving him first with fluffy rice. But now let's talk about Tah, Chin another kind of Tah - Dig which is also a very famous Persian rice dish.

As I said Perhaps Iranian fighting over Tah–Dig ended up with inventing Tah (bottom) Chin (layers). It's Tah–Digey all over and it's enough for everyone on the table to enjoy taste to Tah–Dig as the process to produce Tah–Chin is somehow to let whole rice in the pot go crispy and crunchy. There is also another story of how Tah–Chin was invented, they say another day court chef made mistake and instead of nice fluffy rice he cooked gluey, mushy rice. He was so scared since king was so tough and picky with the food he was served , and always expected the best.

Suddenly this came to chef mind, he can turn gluey rice to a new Tah–Digey dish which King loves. So he mixed gluey rice with yogurt, eggs, saffron and layered in pot with chicken pieces in the middle and latter when it was ready with lots of crunch chef served it with fried saffron barriers on top for garnish. And it was when Tah (Bottom) Chin (layers) was invented.

Not so bad to put fear in your chef isn't it.

Method

For cooking Tah–Dig you cook your normal rice and give it a longer low heat cooking time when your rice is nicely cooked leave it in very low heat for extra 20-30 minutes.

I didn't give you preap and cooking time above as I said when your any kind of rice is ready add 20-30 extra minutes on very low heat and your rice Tah–Dig is ready by then.

But if you want other sorts of Tah–Dig like flat bread, thin slices of potato… it's different process. As I said earlier cooking Persian rice is a different and unique way for cooking rice as they soak the rice two hours before cooking with salt and water. Then in medium size pan and on normal high heat and 1/3 of pot should be filled with water once the water in pot started boiling they add soaked rice to the hot boiling water in the pot. Once the rice is half cooked but not totally soft you drain it with cold water on top that gives a hot rice a shock and rice receiving cold water stats growing longer which leads it a more fluffy texture in cooked rice.

Leave two table of spoons vegetable oil, 1/2 teaspoon brewed saffron for better colour in your Tah–Dig (optional) and if you didn't have saffron add 1/2 teaspoon of turmeric. Then add your thin flat bread spread it nice and even on the pot as it covers all corners of the pot.

Bring back drained rice on top of flat bread on bottom of your pot.

Make a big hole on the middle of your rice to let steam out and add 1/2 glass of hot water with 1 medium spoon of gee or butter or simply vegetable oil , put the lid back on pot tightly.

Leave heat on medium high for 10 minutes and then turn on low for 35 minutes. Once your rice is well soft and fluffy leave on very low heat for extra 15-20 more minutes. Do not open the lid at all while rice it's cooking, opening the lid makes the heat in pot lose its balanced for requiring heat.

For any other sorts of Tah–Dig you do exactly the same like thin layers of sliced potatoes in length, thin layer of beetroot, lettuce leaves for rice with herbs or else you do exactly the same for what you did with flat bread. But if Persian style cooking is so hard for you, you can just use your rice cooker.

If you like to let it go crispy you can by leaving it on heat longer than usual and just add more oil or butter while rice is cooking. This is for rice Tah–Dig but again if you like other kind of Tah–Dig it's not a big problem once your rice in your rice cooker is half cooked transfer it to another pot , wash your rice cooker and add oil or gee in bottom of your rice cooker and then flat bread or else again transfer your half cooked rice to the rice cooker and let the normal rice cooking process happen.

Once your rice cooked an if it turned off before crisp happen turn it on again for few more time after nearly 45 min starting from the beginning of the process your rice and your Tah–Dig is ready for a big crispy crunch. I should mention one thing is very important for best Tah–Chin or even best Tah–Dig specially for beginners its better to use nonstick pot .

Although it's possible to bring it to the right point without nonstick pot but it's less risky if you use a Teflon pot or any other nonstick pot.

For all sorts of Persian dish with rice is best to use long- grain Basmati rices excepts for those sorts of Ash (Persian soup) you can use short grain rices for Ash too as it will fall apart because for Ash always other grains including rice should be cooked on very low heat while it's floating in water or broth and that leads to loose mushy rice which is best only for Ash.

That means for cooking any kind of Ash (Persian soup) No need for rice to save it's nice fluffy shape as it will and should fall apart completely in Ash.

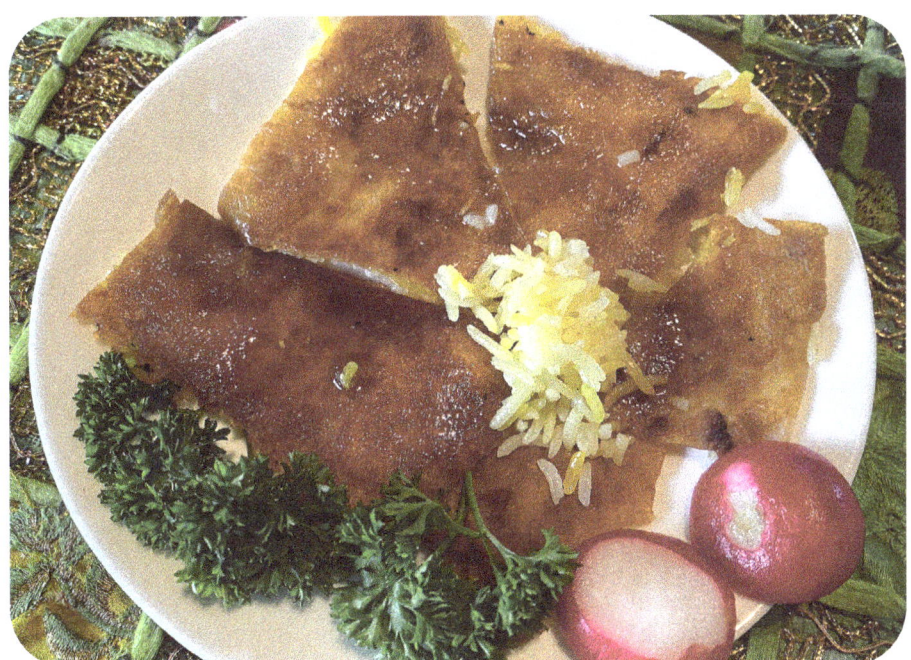

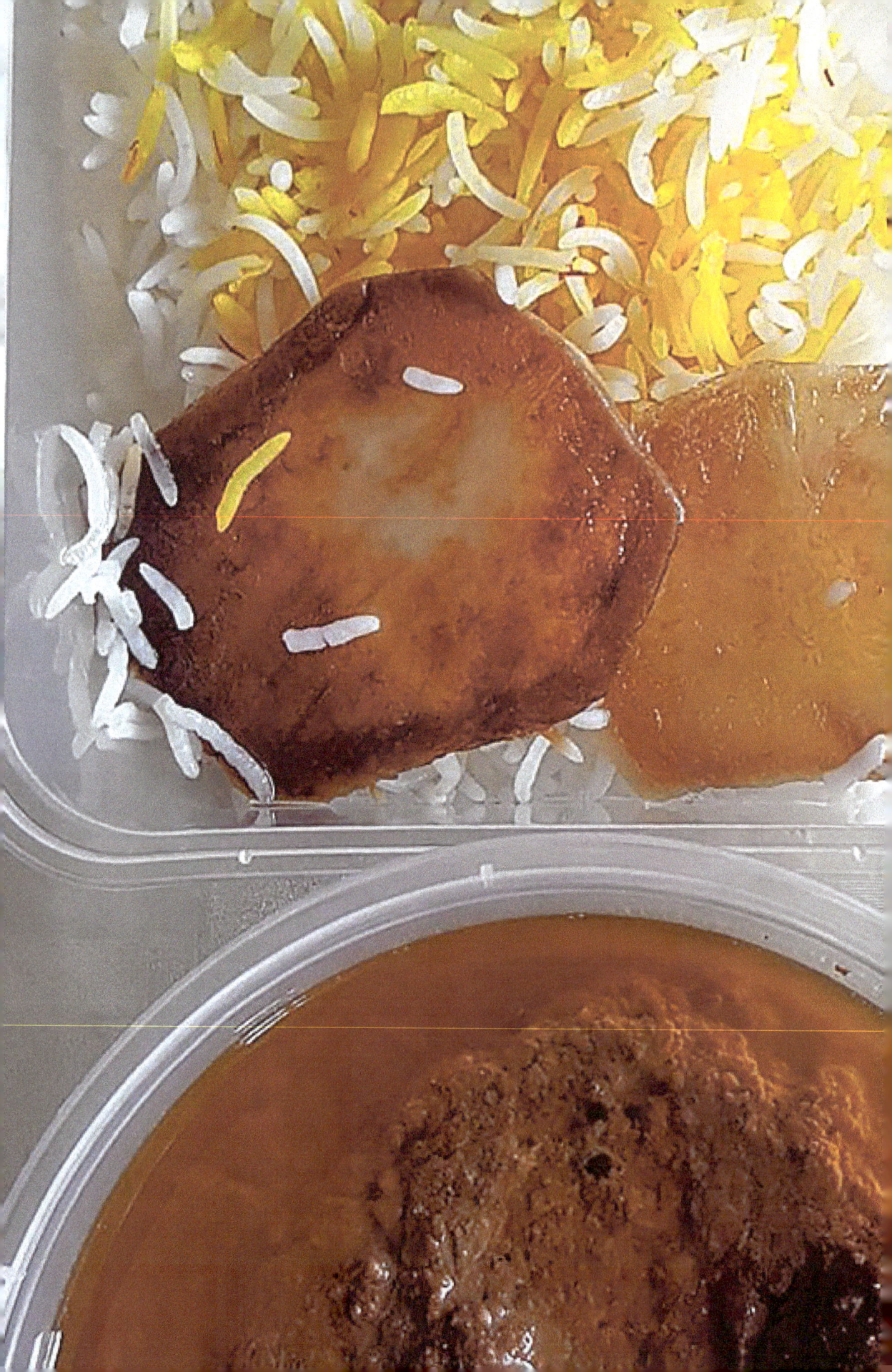

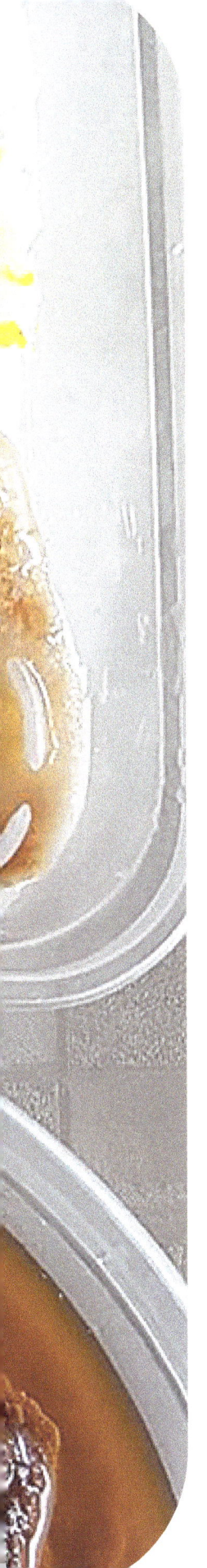

Fesenjoon

Last but not least – Fesenjoon – one of the most luxurious Persian foods. There is never a wedding ceremony in Iran that doesn't serve Fesenjoon.

The taste and appearance might seem strange to people with no idea about this food, but from the very first taste, they fall in love with it.

If you're ever invited to a Persian family home and they serve you with Fesenjoon, this means they care a lot about you. Considering today's economic crises all over the world, including Iran, not many people can afford to serve Fesenjoon to their guests these days, but it's still always served at formal ceremonies and on on weddings tables.

The reputation of Fesenjoon goes back to almost to the beginning of Iran's history, nearly 30,000 years ago. Originating from the north of Iran, as this dish's hero ingredients were grown mostly in the north, however now, it's so famous that it's cooked all over the country. In northern Iran, Fesenjoon is cooked in a special clay pot called a Gamaj, as it is believed the clay pot serves the taste and ingredients much better. In some areas, it is only cooked in a copper pot, but using a Gamaj is more common.

Fesenjoon can be cooked either with chicken or meatballs, but it used to be cooked only with the hunted meats of wild birds, such as pheasants or turkeys. In the old days, hunting in the jungles was very popular, and was considered one of main occupations for men living in wild nature. Another main ingredient is pomegranate molasses, the colour of which is very important to create up a very good and classic Fesenjoon.

Sometimes, a piece of iron or clean horseshoe made of iron is added while the food is cooking to get to the desired colour.

In that case, a great Fesenjoon turns to a very dark stew and maybe this is why it is sometimes called black stew in northern Iran (or maybe because the pomegranate molasses made from wild pomegranate trees has a very dark colour). It is also believed that when iron is added to the pot, the elements released from the iron are good for your health.

Even in the old days, Fesenjoon used to be considered one of the most luxurious foods. There is proverbial saying about someone who is really wealthy that says he eats Fesenjoon every night.

If you check old Persian cookbooks, they will say there are ten different kinds of Fesenjoon, with ten different colours, but these days people are only familiar with one kind of Fesenjoon. For each of these ten versions – some with zucchini, others with fried eggplant – different main ingredients played the hero ingredient – but there was always pomegranate molasses, well-grounded walnuts and meat. In some versions, carrots or even dried almond were used with walnuts.

Fesenjoon is in a category of stews which in ancient food language were called Mosama. Mosama referred to stews with a heavy amount of frying or good amount of oil in it. These days, not many people call stews Mosama. Like everywhere in the world, new generations have brought new styles and usages for words, and new vocabulary is used and is more commonly.

Fesenjoon is also very famous for being one of the most-time consuming Iranian foods. They say a good Fesenjoon comes only from being cooked overnight. It is believed the right taste or colour is only achieved if the ingredients marry together over a very low heat, like a candle, but we all know our modern lifestyles don't allow us to use up so much time just to cook a dish – even if it's Fesenjoon.

Serves 4

Cooking time: 2 hours 30 minutes (or could be more if on very low heat)

- 4 cups walnut, well grounded
- 6 pieces boned, skinless chicken thighs (or other parts if desired)
- 1 tsp turmeric
- 4 tbsp vegetable oil or olive oil
- 1 large onion, finely chopped
- 4 cups pomegranate juice
- 1/4 cup of good quality pomegranate molasses (add more during cooking if you feel it needs more, depending on your taste)
- 1/4 tsp well powdered saffron, brewed with ice or 2 tbsp of boiling water
- 2 tbsp sugar (optional, if you like a sweet taste in this stew – if not, the pomegranate molasses taste would be enough
- Pomegranate seeds and slivered pistachios or almonds for garnish
- Plain long grain basmati rice, to serve

Method

Roast walnuts on direct heat or in the oven until light brown in colour. If cooking on the stove, stir occasionally. Set aside to cool.

In a large bowl, season the chicken with turmeric and half a teaspoon of black pepper and half a teaspoon of salt. Set aside.

In medium pan, fry chicken on both sides until you get a light colour. Add one glass of water and leave on a low heat until the chicken is cooked well. Set aside.

In a food processor, grind the roasted walnut as finely as possible.

Add two cups of pomegranate juice until you get a smooth paste.

In a another medium pot, add the rest of the pomegranate juice, pomegranate molasses and two cups of water. Add the walnut and pomegranate paste, and cook on a very low heat. Stir frequently but not constantly, for at least two hours. Whenever you feel the sauce starting to stick, add two cups of water. (As the sauce cooks, it will start to thicken and change to a deep dark brown colour – the level of darkness in this stew strongly refers to the quality of the pomegranate molasses.)

Add saffron and adjust seasonings (to sweeten, add two tablespoons of sugar, otherwise add a pinch of salt. If you like a stronger taste of pomegranate molasses add more – the original taste is between sweet and sour taste.)

Now add chicken until it starts to fall off the bone, and let it simmer, uncovered, for another 45 minutes on a very low heat. (The right level of heat is important since the sauce must thicken but shouldn't stick to the pot, so whenever you felt it starting to stick to the pot, add a splash of water to prevent the stew from burning.)

Once the sauce is thickened, add to a serving dish. (To keep your chicken from falling apart, serve the chicken pieces out first, and then add sauce on top.) Garnish with pomegranate seeds and slivered almonds and pistachios.

Serve with plain saffron rice and Noosh e Jan (Bon apétit)!

Food for weddings and formal ceremonies

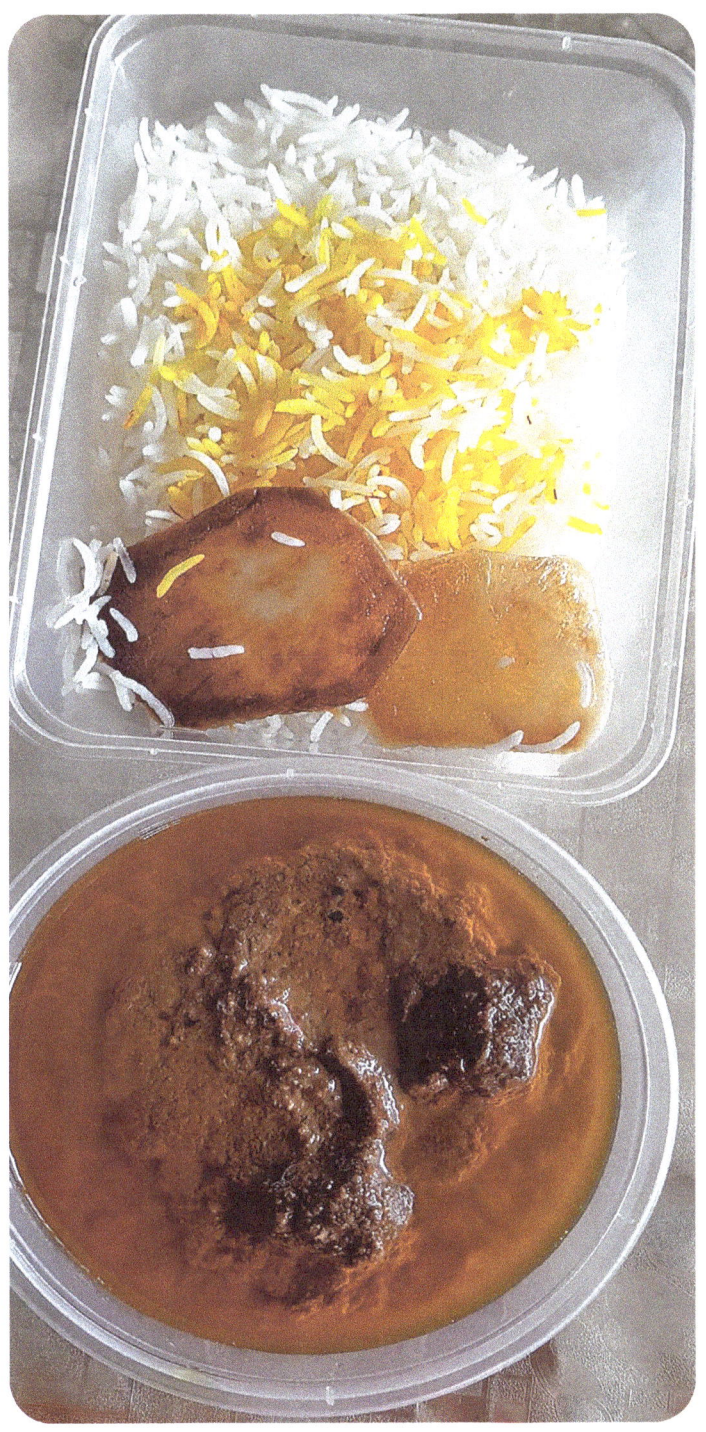

207

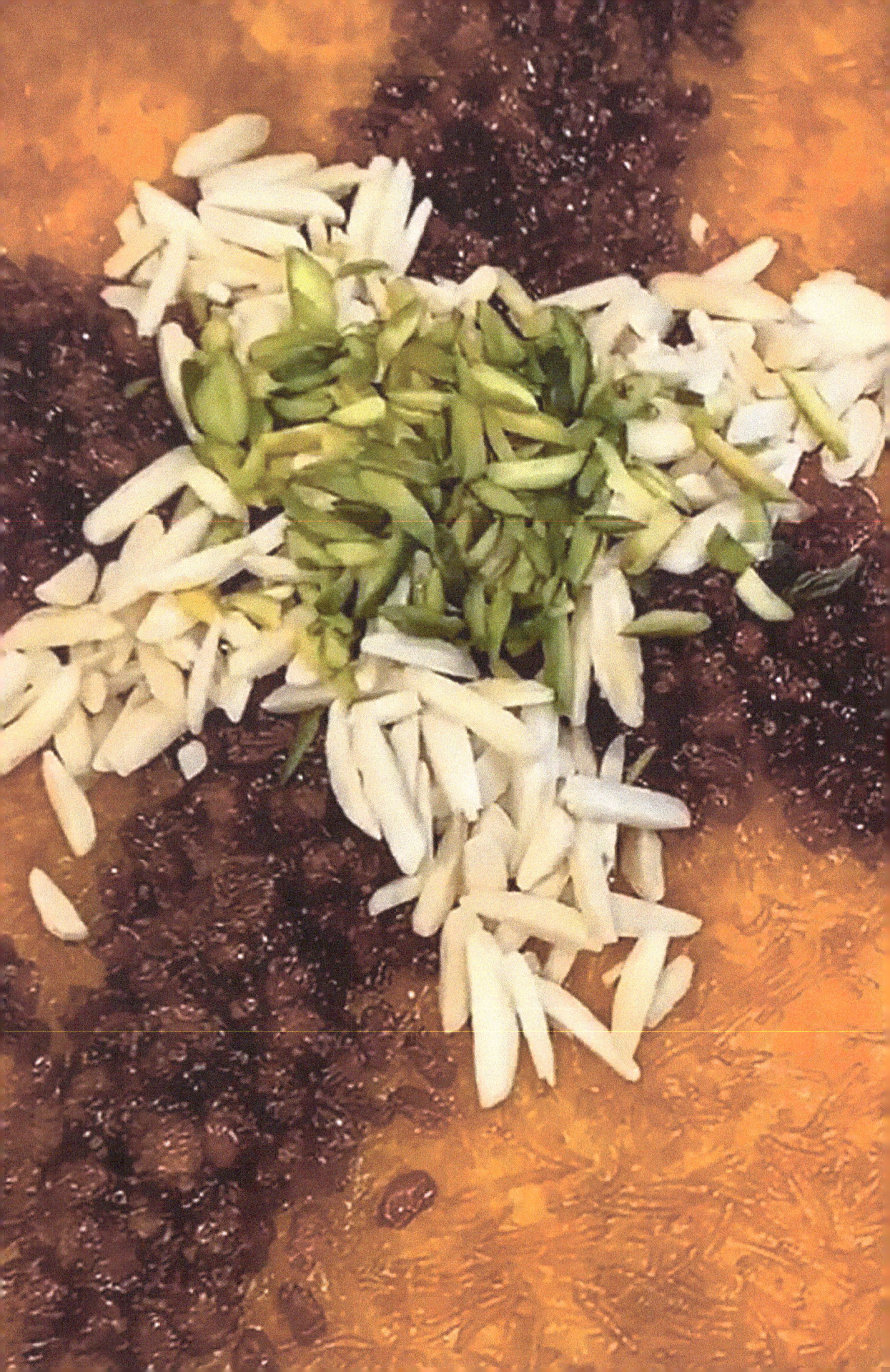

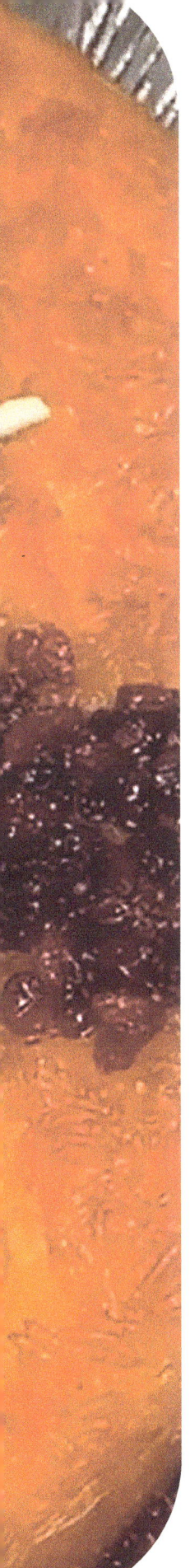

Tah-Chin

Although the variety of food served in wedding and formal ceremonies are so huge but here I pointed to the most common one.

Like every other food for each state, there are also special kinds of cuisine served in formal ceremonies, but these few are always served in every wedding and formal ceremonies. Other cuisines which are definitely very common and famous, depending on many different things such as place, occasion, how well is the host's financial position will be served. And not mentioning their name doesnt mean they are not popular and tasty.

For last cuisine in this category according to my knowledge is Tah–Chin.

I already gave you some information about Tah–Chin. It's story and origin and here is more about this heavenly tasty food.

Tah (bottom) Chin (layers) There is no wedding dinner or formal ceremonies table with Tah–Chin missing on their menu.

- It's looks like in any formal ceremonies Tah–Chin is the proud of the table and for host it's to prove this how a real formal Persian serving should be.

- You can absolutely find no one who doesn't like it, although in formal ceremonies it's not pleasant to bring that noise out of crunch but everyone is so involved with its taste and flavour, I doubt others keep an ear to hear the noise from the crunch.

- So if your invited to a formal persian ceremony and there is lots of Tah–Chin on the table do not afraid of the noise your going to make in every bite of this crunchy creature, because everyone else is doing the same and no one will blame you for that.

- Iranian love for Tah–Dig as I said earlier ended to creating a new dish called Tah–Chin which is Tah Digey all over and in every corner.

- It's a crispy saffron rice stuffed with chicken and fried barberries on top as garnish, although it's possible to skip fried barberries on top but it gives a sensational appearance yet amazing taste to Tah–Chin when added on top.

- I already told you Tah–Chin story and how it was added to Persian cuisine list.

- It's looks like a cake at the end if the baking process process is done correctly but not a sweet cake instead it has that savoury texture.

- The crunch that you get from Tah–Chin is arguably best part of it.

- It goes very well with all sorts of salad specially with any sour taste in salad.

Serving: 4-6

Prep time: 1 1/2 hour

Cooking time: minimum 1 1/2 hour

- 1 and 1/2 cups of thick Greek yogurt
- 2 teaspoon of turmeric

- 2 tablespoons of salt plus 1/2 more for seasoning onion and chicken
- 2 tablespoons of freshly squeezed lemon juice
- 2 medium onion, one grated and set aside and rest thinly sliced
- 3-4 piece of boneless, skinless chicken meat (preferred parts ideally chicken tights)
- 1 cup vegetable oil
- 75 grams of butter
- 3 cups of long grain basmati rice
- 2 eggs
- 1 and 1/2 teaspoon crushed saffron threads brewed with 1/4 cup of hot boiling water or brewed with 4 medium ice cubes (either one of these two ways is used for brewing crushed saffron to boost colour and flavour out of saffron threads)

Method

In a shallow mixing bowl combine 2 tablespoons of yogurt, 1 teaspoon of turmeric, 1 teaspoon of salt and 1 tablespoons of lemon juice with grated onion marinade chicken and leave for at least 1 hour.

Later cook marinated chicken on a very low heat with 1 glass of water. Once chicken is well cooked turn the heat off and leave it until it's completely cool down. Now shredded the chicken roughy in medium size chunks and set aside.

In a medium size pan fry the thin sliced onion with two tablespoons of vegetable oil and season it with salt and continue on frying until sliced onion starts getting soft and colour turn to golden, stir frequently to stop from burning once you get to nice and shiny golden colour turn off the heat and add to shredded cooked chicken and together give a nice mix on low heat for 10 more minutes, then get off the heat and set aside.

If the mixture looks very dry splash drops of water but not too much.

In another medium pot add 3 cups of water, rice, 2 tablespoons of salt, bring these two to boil over high heat and when rice grain are no longer crunchy outside (check occasionally it should still be crunchy inside and not crunchy outside, it needs a bite of experience if this method is hard for you simply use rice cooker for each cup of rice add 1/2 cup of water and for all add 1 tablespoons of salt and two tablespoons of vegetable oil. Let cook like any other normal plain rice you normally cook in rice cooker, like when water is absorbed in rice cooker time to turn off the rice cooker as in this stage rice should not be cooked completely).

For cooking in the pot with straining, when rice is half cooked which rice grains are cooked outside but still crunchy inside time to drain whole rice and add cold water on top, let all extra water drop completely from strainer.

In another large mixing bowl add rest of the yogurt, 1 teaspoon of salt, eggs, brewed saffron, 3 tablespoons of vegetable oil and 1 tablespoons of left lemon juice and whisk eggs with a fork continue until eggs beaten well enough in yogurt.

Continue on whisking the mixture until you see the consistency and now add all drained half cooked rice or rice from rice cooker with this mixture and with a wooden spoon give gentle mix until all the yogurt mixture will cover every grains of rice in the bowl and in every sides each rice grains is covered with mixture very well.

Turn the oven and preheat the oven on 450 degrees.

Spray oven tray or baking pan with vegetable oil or simply brush, it might be best to use is cup cake baking tray as you can have for each person one but the other above moulds are also good. Leave a baking paper underneath.

Add 1/2 mixture and spread it evenly in each side, add shredded cooked chicken with fried onion , spread on top of the mixture evenly, add the rest of mixture on top and spread very evenly.

Add few pieces of cube sized butter in different spots of the pan. All the mixture should be covering the baking pan on all sides nicely in all 4 corners if it's a baking tray.

Whatever mould yours is cover it with aluminium foil, poke the foil with a fork in few different spots to take th extra steam out.

Leave in preheated oven for 1 hour on 450 degree.

Turn the tray a few times so the heat will heat the mixture in all corners and sides.

Gently check few times for when corners looks crusty it time to take out.

While you leave tray out to cool down a bit you can prepare garnish.

Optional:

Fry for 30 seconds:

1/2 cup of washed and drained barberries with 1/2 tablespoons of sugar, 1 tablespoons of brewed saffron.

Take out aluminium foil, leave a serving dish on top of the tray and gently flip over the tray on serving dish like what you always do for flipping over cakes.

Add fried barberries with silvered pistachios on top and time to enjoy.

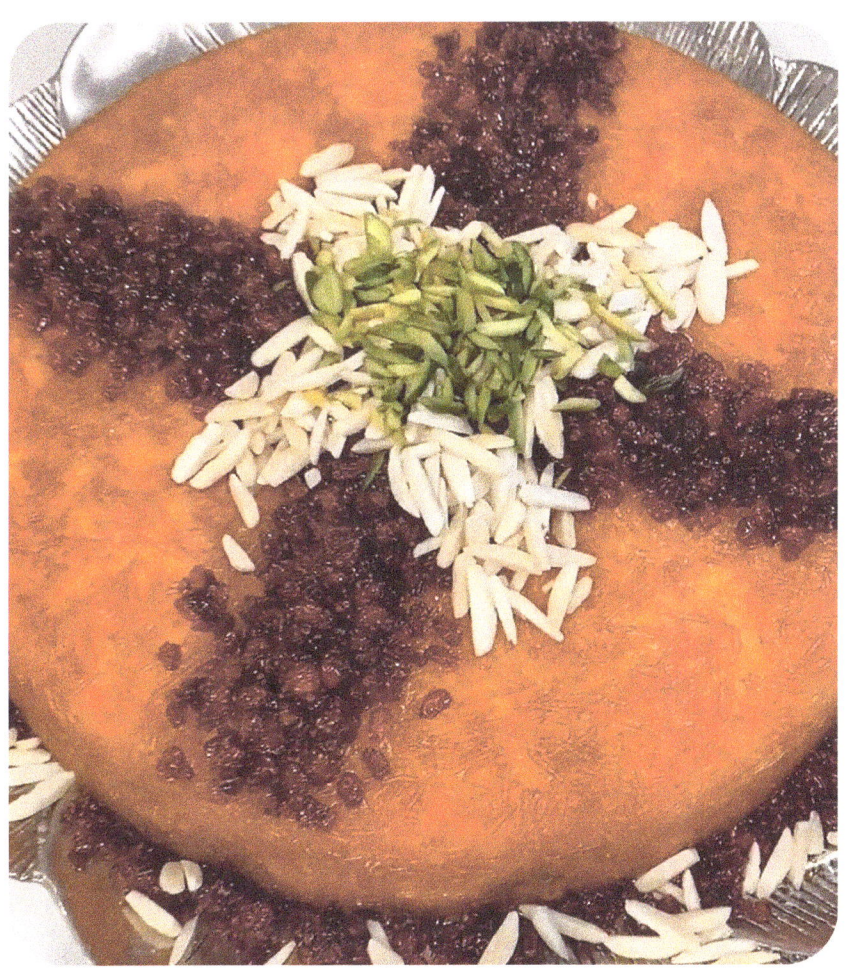

Well, as the Iranian poet says, the book is finished but the story remains.

Which means that there are thousands more Persian recipes, but in this book I just wanted to introduce not only Persian food but the history and traditions behind the most common and well-known Persian foods.

I sincerely hope this book helps people to be introduced to the Iranian culture and traditions even just a little bit, to correct the false media about Iran and Iranians.

We love having guests and we enjoy serving more than being served. If you don't believe me, just find a Persian friend in the community, ask them to cook you one of these dishes and come back to me with the result …

We Iranians have another proverb which says, 'The writing may not be perfect, but please remember that English is my second language. This book is about the love of cooking. I hope you share that love.'

THANK YOU, THANK YOU

I would like to thank the following friends for helping me make this dream come true.

Stephanie Lightfoot for her amazing editing.

With your talent in editing this could have never happened.

Marjorie Tenchaves and welcome merchant team for all their generosity and brave support.

I would also like to thank the following talented friends of mine in helping me capture the photos of my recipes:

Giti Jafari

Raheleh Rezaei

Faeezeh Rafati

Mamma Shookoh catering

Shahnaz Daghagheleh

Neda Bazyariyan

Azadeh Arzhangi

www.ingramcontent.com/pod-product-compliance
Lightning Source LLC
Chambersburg PA
CBHW042358280426
43661CB00096B/1153